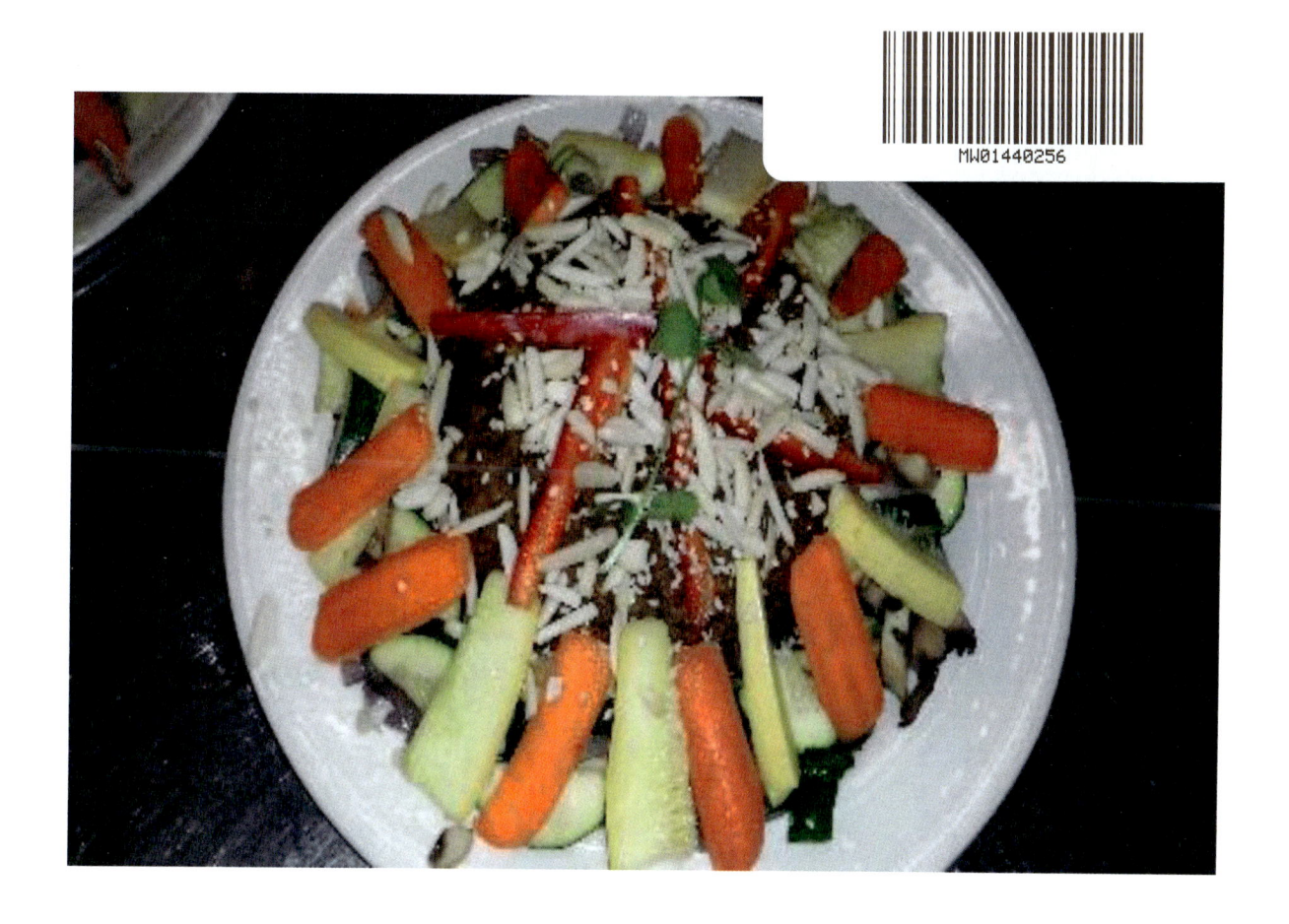

The Wholesome
Vegan-Gluten-free
Gourmet Cook Book

Phil Kvasnica

The Wholesome Vegan-Gluten-free Gourmet Cook Book

January 2020
Author and editor: Phil Kvasnica
Knowledgeable contributors, influences and inspiration:
        Genesis 1:29, et al (Bible)
        Juli Griffith (friend & director of local celiac group)
        living-foods.com
        rawfoods.com
        Nomi Shannon
        David Wolfe
        Creative Health Institute(chi.com, formerly Ann Wigmore Institute, Union City, Michigan)
        <u>Prescription for Nutritional Healing</u> (James & Phyllis Balch)
        Mani Niall, natural baker, Los Angeles, CA (<u>Sweet & Natural Baking</u>)
        <u>The Raw Truth</u>, (Jordan Rubin)
        Cousins raw cuisine café & culinary school (recipes)
        Dr. Richard Schulze (American Botanical Pharmacy)
        and many others (see also Bibliography)

Cover photo: Photo courtesy of Connor Roche; "vegetarian" meal (actually vegan, gluten-free) made by author for 5 hotel banquet guests, "Mount Curry" (see in "Beans, Rice & Grains" section) Incidentally, the author's job as a hotel banquet cook has contributed to several other recipes in this book.

Author's Note

Author's background: 7th grade was the first time I knew something was wrong. While in class, all of a sudden, my nose "erupted" with all this yellow mucus, so I was wiping it on my clothes, and one of my classmates said to go to the bathroom and clean up. Later on, for some reason, I found that I was getting headaches & nasty or depressed moods after eating wheat foods. After adjusting my diet & experimenting with all sorts of alternative foods, and having been formally tested at the Olive Garvey Center for Health in Wichita, Kansas, I found out the "truth", that my body did indeed have a noticeable reaction to wheat and dairy, as well as a few other foods & ingredients which I now avoid as much as possible. Being a hotel cook requires some testing of foods, but other than that, my current diet is at least 95% gluten-free and dairy-free. I buy most of my specialty groceries at the local food co-op, buy natural juices & basically eat rice, beans & veggies for dinner. Often I'll eat at the local salad bar. After all, the body does work better with live enzymes, and fresh fruits & vegetables are a great way to get them. As for being vegan, I figured that as long as I was avoiding lactose & casein, I might as well avoid E. coli, salmonella, and all those other nasty bacteria by not eating meat either. So, like I said, I'm still 95% vegan and gluten-free. Besides, wheat is insoluble fiber, which pushes everything out of your colon like a bulldozer, which would be good, if you ate something poison. Rice, on the other hand, is easily digestible, and legumes (beans, lentils, peas, etc.), in spite of the gas, are a great source of protein, and complement the proteins in rice. I'm not saying wheat is an "unhealthy grain", because it is otherwise rich in nutrients. When they leave the nutrients in, (germ, bran and all), that is. Food processors have a nasty confusing habit of taking all the good stuff out of the grain, and selling it cheaper, then selling the good stuff as separate ingredients for high prices. Apparently they don't realize that all that milling is costing them money which they may or may not recover with what they charge for the "adulterated" products. All in the name of job security. I have also stopped eating so many other "fake foods" such as white sugar, white flour, etc., because, obviously, they aren't complete(not to mention not very appetizing.) And whose erroneous idea was it to put white rice flour in gluten-free flour? This milling mistake has been going on since at least 1950 or earlier. Thank God for co-ops, even though some of them sell that junk, most are whole-foods focused, which is how God made the foods in the first place. Read Genesis 1:29, 3 John 2, and John 10:10 in the Bible. That's probably why people living in Tahiti are so healthy. Think about that one. Simplicity. Time to get out of our "cheapskate" mentality and pursue "quality" and "real."

Author's professional and related experience:
10 years in various forms of the food industry:(not including family meals)
    Restaurants (full-service, fast-food, buffet)
    Hotels
    Banquet service
    School Food Services (school district, university, vocational)
    Mass Food Production (military)
    Culinary school graduate
    Finished "cum laude" from Nutrition Specialist program (Ashworth Univ.)
    Training in organic farming practices (Dr. Rhonda Janke, KSU)
20 years of focusing on eating more wholesome, wheat-free, dairy-free, animal-free, simple (minimally-processed) foods, and as a result, being "too healthy" to require trips to the doctor for various ailments, and also avoiding any further potentially harmful vaccinations of questionable content.

Table of Contents

	Page
Table of Contents	
Purpose of this Book	1
Preface	2
Measurement & Conversions	3
Cooking Basics	4
Equipment & Utensils Needed	7
Amino Acids, Brain & Healing Foods	8
Omega Fatty Acids	10
Produce (by COLOR)	11
Herbs & Spices	16
Reputed Healing Herbs	19
General Produce	20
Flavors of the World	27
RECIPES:	
Appetizer Prep Tips	28
Appetizers	29
5-layer guacamole dip	29
Fluted stuffed mushrooms	29
Funghi con pinoli(stuffed mushrooms)	29
Potato Wedges	30
Spinach-Artichoke Dip	30
Stuffed Cabbage	30
Stuffed Peppers	31
Ukrainian Xlopse(stuffed cabbage)	31
Beans, Rice & Grains Prep Tips	32
Beans, Rice & Grains	34
Adzuki & Jasmine Rice Pilaf	34
Asian Rice	34
Best Rice & Vegetable Pilaf	35
Goddess Lentils & Spinach Pilaf	35
Honey-Mustard Rice Pilaf	36
Jambalaya	36
Italian Vegetable Risotto	37
Lemon-Ginger Lentils	37
Mincemeat Breakfast Cereal	38
Mount Curry Lentil Pilaf	38
Thai Peanut Satay	39
Potassium Potpourri	39
Raspberry-Spice Buckwheat Granola	40
Red Beans & Rice Crockpot-Style	40
Red Lentil Curry Masala	40
Red Quinoa & Lentils with Stir-fry Vegetables	41
Rice & Bean Vegetable Pilaf	41
Rice Pilaf, Sheraton (Daughters of Amer. Revolution)	42
Rosemary-Red Onion Polenta	42
Supergrain & Fruit Cereal for a month	43
Taco-Rice Casserole	43
Tahini Peanut Satay	44
Vegan/Vegetarian Thanksgiving Dinner	44
World Traveler Rice Pilaf	45
Wednesday 7/10/13 Dinner	45
Beverages	46
Curative Power Tea	46
Fen Beer	46
Fruit Drink	46
Macho Man's Booster Iced Tea	46
Pina Colada	47
Red Tea	47

Table of Contents

Strong Drink for Toxic People	47
Summer Fruit Jazz	48
Breads	49
Gluten-Free New Bread	49
GF Seed Bread idea	49
Hearty Hazelnut Bread	50
Dense Fruit & Nut Bread (unleavened)	50
Bread Mixes	51
Breakfast Food Possibilities	52
Cakes	53
Black Forest Fruit & Spice Cake	53
Black Forest Cake	53
Carrot Spice Marble Cake	54
Chocolate Cake (GF-Vegan revision)	55
Happy Fruit Cake	55
Tantalizing Torte Chilled Layer Cake	56
Black Forest Bundt-Brownie	56
Cookies, Muffins & Pancakes	57
Blueberry Muffins	57
Buckwheat-Blueberry-Maple Nut Pancakes	57
Carob-Date Confection (Raw Donut Holes)	58
Ginger-Molasses Monster Cookies	59
Happy Cookies	59
Maple Pecan Sandies	60
Mom's Corn Muffins	60
Phil's Chocolate Chip Cookies	60
Quinoa Flake Cookies	61
Seven-Layer Bars (Coconut-Pecan bars)	61
Sesame Cookies	61
Desserts, Candy & Pudding	62
Apple-Cinnamon-Caramel Sauce/Syrup	62
Baklava (GF, raw revision)	62
Chocolate Pizza	63
Carobbean Fruit Parfait	63
Cookies & Cream Pudding idea	63
Mulled Blueberry Pudding	64
Pistachio Pudding	64
Rhubarb Fruit Crisp	64
Gourmet Rice Krispie Bars	65
Rosehip Syrup	65
Streudel for Fruit Crisp (Sheraton)	65
Sweet Peach Chutney	65
Whipped Topping-natural (idea)	66
Wild Rice Pudding (instead of white rice pudding)	66
Egg/Meat/Cheese/Wheat Alternatives	67
Eggless Cornbread Quiche	67
Parmesan cheese	67
Breakfast Sausage Blend	67
Pasta & Pizza	68
Borscht Lasagna	68
GF Vegan Vegetable Lasagna	68
Linguini Alfredo Primavera	69
Pasta Primavera	69
Phil's Pasta Salad (Sheraton)	69
Penne Garden Pasta Salad	70
Quinoa Alfredo Primavera	70
Quinoa Pasta Salad	70
Spelt Pizza (revision)	71
Traditional Lasagna	72

Table of Contents

Pies & Tarts — 73
GF, DF~ Chocolate Pie — 73
Pecan Pie — 73
Turtle Pie — 73
Pickles, Relish, Salsa & Sauce — 74
Black Bean & Corn Relish — 74
Afterburner Untomato Salsa — 74
Chili Verde Salsa — 74
Coconut Milk Sauce — 74
Medium Salsa — 75
Medium Untomato Salsa — 75
Mom's Zucchini Relish — 75
Pesto — 75
Pesto Cream Sauce — 75
Pickles — 76
Pickled Red Onions & Cucumbers — 76
Pico de Gallo — 76
Salsa Blanca — 76
Souped-up Black Bean & Corn Relish — 77
Super Hot Sauce — 77
Salads & Dressings — 78
Ambrosia Salad — 78
Asian Dish — 78
Asian Slaw — 78
Asian Salad-Indian version — 79
Beans-n-Greens Salad — 79
Curried Bean Salad — 80
4-Pepper Mexican Salad — 80
Gourmet Tropical Salad — 81
Gratest Salad — 81
Indian Salad — 82
Italian Leek Salad — 82
Mediterranean Salad — 82
Mint-Apple Kiwi Salad — 83
Mexican Tortilla Casserole — 83
Mextravaganza — 83
Mini Mexican Salad — 84
Oblivion Salad — 84
Pedro's Garden — 85
Penne Garden Pasta Salad — 85
Piquant Mustard Potato Salad (Sheraton) — 85
Rainbow Vegetable Salad — 86
Salad with Almonds & Sprouts — 86
Salad for a King — 86
Salad with Pesto & Pizzazz — 87
Salad — 88
Spinach Salad — 88
Summer Fruit Jazz — 88
Super Salad (Salad bar) — 89
The Salad Bar — 89
Tropical Tango Fruit Salad — 90
Ukrainian Beet Salad — 90
#1 Honey Mustard Dressing — 90
Creamy Fiesta Honey-Mustard Dressing — 90
Green Goddess Dressing — 91
Honey-Mustard Dressing — 91
Sweet & Tangy Raspberry Vinaigrette — 91
Raspberry-Grapeseed Oil Vinaigrette — 91
Phil's Famous Yogurt Dressing — 92

Table of Contents

Smoothies — 93
  Basic — 93
  #2 Superfruit Basic — 93
  #3 Pomegranate-Acai Treat — 93
  #4 Digestive Dynamo — 93
  #5 Enzyme-Vita-Meister — 93
  General Ingredient Possibilities — 94

Soups & Stews — 95
  Borscht — 95
  Butternut Squash Stew — 95
  Cold Annihilating Soup — 95
  Corn Chowder — 96
  Creole Southern Gumbo — 96
  German Cabbage & Apples (Sheraton) — 96
  Hearty Cold-Day Soup — 97
  Gumbo — 97
  Hash — 98
  Melon Soup — 98
  Mexican Minestrone — 99
  Minestrone-Sweet Potato Savoy — 99
  Minestrone-Butternut Squash & Mushroom — 100
  Potato Soup — 100
  Spicy Vegetarian Chili — 101
  Vegetable-Bean Stew — 101
  Vegetable Potato Soup — 102

Vegetables — 103
  Chef School Stir-Fry — 103
  Creole Dinner — 103
  East-Indian Shepherd's Pie — 104
  Endive & Lentils with Sunchoke Sauce — 104
  Mexican Mojo — 105
  Potato Curry — 105
  Potato Pancakes — 105
  Quinoa-Beet Curry — 106
  Spinach Vindaloo Curry — 106
  Sweet Potato with Quinoa Pasta — 107
  Sweet Potatoes with Wild Rice — 107
  Sweet Curry Masala Vegetable Stir-fry — 108
  Veggie Stir-fry for KSU Day Lily Club (Sheraton) — 108

Recipes For Reformulation — 109
Various Miscellaneous Diets — 110
Recipe Costing-Salads & Dressings - Example — 111
Bibliography & Recommended Reads — 112

Appendix
  Commentary Preface — C1
  1) Fat, Sick & Starved People — C2
  2) Balanced Alternatives — C3
  3) Piecemeal Healthy Foods — C4
  4) Junk in Food — C5
  5) Monopoly of Certain Foods — C6
  6) Politics & Celebrities — C7
  7) Conventional vs. Healthy — C8
  8) Nutrition--Animal-based food — C9
  9) Health-related Surgeries-$$K — C10
  10) Countless Diseases from **S**tandard **A**merican **D**iet — C11
  11) Healthy Foods, Big Appetites — C12
  12) Calories and Sugars 101 — C13
  13) Well-being vs. Healthcare — C14

Table of Contents

Nutritional Content of Foods
Nutrition-Fruits
Nutrition-Grains
Nutrition-Vegetables
Nutrition-Legumes
Nutrition-Nuts, Seeds & Oils
Nutrition-Herbs & Spices

Purpose of this Book

Note to Readers:

~~All recipes in this book are, by principle, gluten-free and dairy-free, and vegan, unless otherwise noted (about 3). The sole purpose of this book is to increase the reader's health and also refresh their love of food with safe alternatives to all the "mystery food" out there, which is produced more from factories, clever marketing techniques, ignorance & political greed than the customer's needs.

~~This book is not focused on any ethnic brand of cooking, but rather "health conscious cooking", since "conventional" cooking is only concerned about dressing things up, for the sake of flavor, nuance, or appearance. Methods such as roasting peppers to burn them, or using traditional roux's, and fancy "French cooking" terms won't dominate this book. What you **will** find is home-style cooking, progressive recipes, and ingredients that may be somewhat unfamiliar, but with an emphasis not only on taste, but on healthy practices, overall well-being, and nutritional content.

The only thing **YOU** have to provide yourself is the quality foods, such as organic, or sustainably-grown foods. We are only teaching you how to prepare the food. While it is true that non-organic foods may have similar nutrients, as they should compared to their organic counterparts, the unnecessary chemicals in the non-organic foods may produce undesirable ills in your body. What's more, the nutritional barrenness of most chemical-laden soils would be of little benefit.

Happy Cooking!/ To your health!

Language	Phrase	Language	Phrase
Afrikaans	Op jou gesondheid	Indonesian	untuk kesehatanmu
Arabian	lasihtuk (iasihatuka)	Irish	do shlainte
Azerbaijani	saglamligin ucun	Italian	Buon appetito
Bangla	Apanara sbasthya	Japanese	kenko no tame ni
Bulgarian	za tvoe zdrave	Korean	dangsin-ui geogang-e
Burmese	sang kyannmarrayyaatwat	Lithuanian	tavo sveikatai
Chinese	Dui ni de jiankang	Malay	untuk kesihatan anda
Czech	Do brow chut!	Nepali	Tapainko svasthyama
Danish	for dit helbred	Portugese	para sua saude
Filipino	sa iyong kalusugan	Romanian	pentru sanatatea ta
French	Bon appetit	Russian	k vashemu zdorov'yu
German	Gesundheit!	Slavic	na zdravii
Greek	stin ygeia sou	Somali	caafimaadl (to your health)
Haitian Creole	pou sante ou	Spanish	a tu salud
Hawaiian	I kou olakino	Swahili	kwa afya yako
Hindi	aapakee sehat ke lie	Swedish	till din halsa
Hungarian	egeszsegedre	Thai	Pheux sukhphaph khxng khun

Purpose of this Book

Preface

Why Another Book on Healthy Recipes?
1) Too many fat, sick and starved people
2) Not enough balanced alternatives to "the usual" food
3) Piecemeal healthy foods, no well-known method of assembly
4) Junk in food (artificial flavors/colors, sweeteners, corn syrups, preservatives, etc.)
5) Monopoly of certain foods to human demise (wheat, dairy, meat, etc.)
6) Too much political- or celebrity-bias in the food industry
7) More focus on conventional ingredients rather than nutritional content
8) Vast epidemic of mal-nutrition and/or over-fed, under-nourished
9) Empty calories, cheap excessively-processed "manufactured" foods
10) Too many animal-"rich", vital-nutrient-poor foods
11) Spraying vitamins & minerals onto foods doesn't work like nature intended
12) Health-related surgeries too expensive
13) We need more people-oriented health, not politics-oriented "health"
14) Animal-based foods are void of dietary fiber, and cause more problems than solutions
15) Dairy allergies, wheat allergies, celiac disease, high cholesterol, diabetes, etc.
16) Negative effects from eating foods which "you're not supposed to eat"
17) Countless diseases and disorders due to our "Standard American Diet"
18) So many "healthy, light, low-calorie" foods that don't satisfy big appetites
19) Calorie confusion (good calories, bad calories, empty calories, 2000 calories,etc.)
20) Well-being vs. "healthcare"
21) More education about wholesome, nutrient-dense foods and how to use them
22) Why not have healthy, guilt-free, satisfying AND delicious food?
23) Alcohol/Wine-free, Dairy-Free, Animal-Free, Wheat-Free, Junk-Free (includes chemicals)
24) Signaling an end to the ubiquitous "sinful dessert", & creating "healthy" (guilt-free) desserts

Measurement Conversions

Cooking Terms Imperial & Metric	Conversions Imperial (English) system used in this book	Example: 1" = 1 inch = 2.54 cm			Metric
c = cup	16 Tbsp	48 tsp	1/2 pint	1 cup	237 mL
qt = quart	32 oz (liquid)	4 cups	2 pints	1/4 gallon	.95 L
gal = gallon	128 oz (liquid)	16 cups	8 pints	4 quarts	3.8 L
tsp = teaspoon	1/6 ounce(liquid)	1/3 Tbsp	1/96 pint	1/48 cup	6 mL
Tbsp = tablespoon	1/2 ounce(liquid)	1/16 cup	1/32 pint	1/64 qt	17mL
oz = ounces	1/16 lb	28.35 g	0.166667		28,350 mg
lb = pounds	16 ounces	1/2000 ton			454g
L = Liter (volume)	33.8 oz	.0001 cubic meters(10cm^3)	1.056 pint	.264 gal.	
mL = milliLiter	.0338 fluid ounce				1 milliliter *
g = gram (weight)	1000 mg	.001 kg	.035oz		
mg = milligram	1/1000 grams	.000035 oz			1000 mcg
kg = kilogram	1000 grams	2.2 lbs			
mcg = microgram	1/1000 milligram	.000000035 oz			
cm = centimeter	.01 meters	.39 inches			
1" = 1 inch	2.54 centimeters		Cups	*Milliliters	Tablespoons
1 tsp	multiply by	42	7/8 cup	210 mL	14
1 tsp	multiply by	36	3/4 cup	180 mL	12
1 tsp	multiply by	31.8	2/3 cup	160 mL	10.6
1 tsp	multiply by	30	5/8 cup	150 mL	10
1 tsp	multiply by	24	1/2 cup	120 mL	8
1 tsp	multiply by	18	3/8 cup	90 mL	6
1 tsp	multiply by	16	1/3 cup	80 mL	5.3
1 tsp	multiply by	12	1/4 cup	60 mL	4
1 tsp	multiply by	6	1/8 cup	30 mL	2
		1 tsp x 3=1 Tbsp x 2 = 1/8 cup	16th cup: add 1 Tbsp		
		1/3 tspx 6=1 Tbsp x 2=1/8 cup			
		1/8 tsp = 1/24 Tbsp			
		1/4 tsp = 1/12 Tbsp			

Teaspoons	Milliliters	ounces (1/8 cup = 1 ounce standard)		
1/8 tsp	5/8 (.625) mL	1/48 oz		
1/4 tsp	1 1/4 (1.25) mL	1/24 oz		
1/3 tsp	1 2/3 (1.67) mL	1/18 oz		
1/2 tsp	2.5 mL	1/12 oz		
1 tsp	5 mL	1/6 oz		
2 tsp	10 mL	1/3 oz		
1/4 Tbsp (1/2 of 1/2 Tbsp)	3.75 mL	1/8 oz		
1/2 Tbsp	7.5 mL	1/4 oz		
3/4 Tbsp	11.25 mL	3/8 oz		
1 Tbsp	15 mL	1/2 oz		
2 Tbsp (1/8 cup)	30 mL	1 oz		

Cooking Basics-General Info

The ingredients at right are not used in the recipes of this book, due to their manufactured nature; it is also recommended that you not add them, or any products that contain them, when you make these recipes, for the benefit of your own health (no matter how "cheap").

Maltodextrin, dextrose, or other similar isolated/manufactured ingredients
artificial colors, flavors, preservatives, etc.
caramel color
MSG, etc.
alcohol, wine, liquor, or other such fermented beverages
white sugar, white flour, white rice, white vinegar
aspartame, sucralose, and other artificial sweeteners
high-fructose corn syrup, corn syrup in general
anything else with no immediate garden or orchard source(mystery ingredients)

Food Preparation Terms

bunch	several single stalks tied together
coarsely-chopped	1/4" - 1/2" size
dash	1 shake of a seasoning
dice (square cube)	square pieces of the same length, height and depth
garnish	the finishing touch on a dish of food. Whole herb, sauce, fruit, nut
julienne	1/8 x 1/8 x 2 inches long up to 1/4 x 1/4 x 2 inches
matchstick cut	1/8 x 1/8 x 1 inch long
quartered	cut in half lengthwise, then cut in half across the width ("+")
sprig	often used for rosemary, parsley, mint, or cilantro: 1 short stalk about 2-4 inches

Butter/Fat Alternatives

avocado, mashed or pureed
banana (ripe)
coconut: milk, flour, oil — coconut oil "okay" for shortening substitute(pie crust, etc.) but melts too quickly
pear puree — x amount of plum puree replaces y amount of fat
plum puree — x amount of plum puree replaces y amount of fat
oil: olive, sunflower, walnut, sesame — 3/4 cup oil replaces 1 cup butter

Dairy & Egg Alternatives

flaxseed — 1/4 cup flaxseed blended with 1/2 cup (1:2 ratio) water for 2 minutes = [1 egg]
alternative: 1/3 cup flaxseed blended with 1 cup water; or 1Tbsp: 3 Tbsp, etc.
applesauce — 1/4 c. applesauce (per egg) can be used as egg replacer (holds things together)
psyllium seed — holds up to 14 times its weight in water, gel-like consistency when moistened
pine nut (a.k.a. pignoli) — taste, color and texture similar to parmesan cheese

Fats & Oils

oil:butter ratio -- 3/4 cup oil for 1 cup butter

olive	extra virgin: salads, soups, etc. refined or "light" used for sautéing or high heat
walnut	almost anything, typically desserts, salads; Omega-3 fatty acids
flax	dressings, thickener, desserts, dietary fiber/oil supplement; Omega-3 fatty acids
almond	desserts(sweet culinary almond oil only), good skin oil
sesame	Asian food. Untoasted flavor is brighter, toasted flavor is richer; Omega-6 EFA's
peanut	Asian foods, deep-fat frying, produces crispy product
Tahini (ground sesame seeds)	Middle-Eastern foods, used as a spread, garnish, dip, sauce, etc.
avocado	using oil in food may overload liver, use avocado fruit in food. Oil good for skin. [7]
sunflower	salad oil, salad dressings/sauces, refrigerator-safe(does not solidify)
macadamia	desserts, cakes, beneficial to skin
apricot	desserts, sweet or baked goods, good for skin
coconut	frying/sauteing, popcorn, baking, soups, melts too fast for pastry, benefits skin
***cottonseed oil**	**NOT USED NOR RECOMMENDED--non-food plant, high pesticide use**

Dry vs. Fresh weights

shiitake mushrooms — 1/2 oz. dried mushrooms = about 6 oz fresh

Gels & Thickening Agents

carrageenan — from Irish moss. Used to thicken juices, sauces, dressings,etc.
agar-agar — used to thicken puddings and gelatin (also used in laboratory petri dishes!)

Cooking Basics-General Info

flax seed	absorbs excess liquid in cooked foods, leavening (egg replacer)
psyllium seed/husk	fiber laxative, can make aspics, holds up to 14x its own weight in water
xanthan gum (1/4 tsp at a time)	Gives gluten-free flours more elasticity and body. Mix thoroughly into flour
arrowroot (Maranta arundinacea)	digestible, thickens bland, low-salt/protein food. Clear "slurry" thickener

Gluten-free baking flours

almond	off-white flour from the famous nut(actually seed of a fruit similar to apricot)
amaranth	light-beige flour from small iron-rich seeds of South American broad-leaf plant
blue corn (chip, tortilla, taco shells)	medium to dark blue "Indian-type" corn with pleasant taste
Bob's Red Mill GF all-purpose	complete baking flour for gluten-free products. Good performance, yellowish
Bob's Red Mill Gar-Fava flour	"garbanzo-fava" flour with other supporting ingredients for good finished product
brown rice flour	somewhat gritty but high in vitamin B and fiber, easily digestible flour
buckwheat	nutritional powerhouse grain, used for buckwheat pancakes. Dark flour
coconut	nut provides juice, milk, flaked or shredded; potassium, good fat; low-glycemic
fava bean	dense flour from large Mediterranean broad bean
Four-flour bean mix (and others)	see Bette Hagman's "The Gluten-Free Gourmet Bakes Bread" (5)
garbanzo(chick pea)	good for cakes, chocolate, spices; flour cooked to overcome "bean" flavor
millet flour	yellow color, rich in B-vitamins, can substitute for rice flour
mung bean flour	sweet flour, good in desserts
pea flour	starchy protein flour, yellow or green. May grind split peas for fresh flour.
quinoa	complete-protein light flour
sorghum	white-colored flour, grain often used for molasses, high carb, low-nutrient
soy flour (light yellow)	complete-protein flour. Adopts flavors
tapioca (Cassava [manioc yuca])	root starch used for pudding, gluten-free flour additive, corn starch substitute
proven gluten-free flour mix	**used in "Carrot-Spice Marble Cake" (see "Cakes")**
yields moist and tender cake,	**10% amaranth flour**
stays together.	**10% sorghum flour**
	40% corn flour
	40% buckwheat flour

White flours for white cake/bread:

coconut	replace up to 100% of wheat flour; add 2-3 eggs (or flax) & extra liquid per 1/2 cup
almond	
sorghum	
amaranth	
white quinoa	

Sweeteners

Agave nectar	nectar from agave plant, used in Tequila. Substitute 3/4 cup Agave per cup sugar
Cane sugar, or turbinado	brown sugar. Preferable over white processed (devitalized) sugar.
Carob powder (Ceratonia siliqua)	roasted locust bean, calcium-rich, similar-flavored caffeine-free cocoa substitute
Chocolate(cacao bean)	blend with cocoa bean-base
Date fines/date sugar	natural "sugar" in the form of finely ground dates, use like brown (cane) sugar
Honey (bee product)	liquefied, solid ("organic"), honeycomb, replace sugar with 1/2 as much honey
Maple syrup/sugar	sweetener from sap of Sugar Maple tree (Acer saccharum). Pancakes, etc.
Molasses, unsulphured	sweet, rich, high-mineral liquid sweetener; cane, beet, sorghum; 1 cup = 12 oz
Stevia	use leaf in tea, or powder (300x sweeter than sugar). Use extract in baked goods
Vanilla bean	long bean from Madagascar, used in ice cream, extract, desserts, flavorings
coconut sugar	caramel-colored granulated sugar

Vinegars

raw apple cider vinegar (Bragg)	("ACV") with "mother" (preferred), herb vinegars, salad dressings, tonic drinks
red wine vinegar	sweet/sour/bitter. salads and sauces both cold and cooked
coconut vinegar	more bitter than apple cider vinegar, has amino acids (nut origin), use on salads
tarragon vinegar	pleasant herbal flavor, made with tarragon herb, used in salads, French foods
rice vinegar	commonly used in Asian foods, herb vinegars, musky fermented-rice flavor

Cooking Basics-General Info

Seasonings & Other Blends	**(courtesy: Frontier Herbs organic herb & spice co.)**
5-spice powder (Asian)	fennel seed, star anise, cloves, cinnamon, white pepper
Cajun (New Orleans)	basil, bay, cayenne, chili powder, cumin, fennel, garlic, marjoram, nutmeg,
Cajun, continued	onion, oregano, paprika, parsley, thyme, sea salt
Chili powder (Mexican, etc.)	cumin, coriander, onion, garlic, chili pepper
Curry (Indian)	turmeric, coriander, cardamom, chilies, cumin, fenugreek, paprika
Dash-o-dill (great on salads, grains)	dill weed, onions, orange peel, garlic
Falafel (Middle East)	corn, chickpeas, onion, garlic, red bell pepper, spinach, tomato, fava beans, salt
Fines Herbes (French)	basil, chervil, chives, marjoram, tarragon
Garam Masala (Indian)	cardamom, cinnamon, cloves, coriander, cumin, mace, bay leaf, black pepper
Gumbo file (Cajun){herbal thickener}	sassafras, thyme
Herbes de Provence (French)	basil, lavender flowers, marjoram, rosemary, savory, tarragon, thyme
Hummus (Middle East)	chickpeas, lemon juice, garlic, onion
Italian seasoning	rosemary, basil, oregano, marjoram, sage, thyme
Pizza seasoning (Italy)	basil, fennel, garlic, onion, oregano, thyme
Thai Seasoning (Thailand)	basil, cayenne, cilantro, coriander, cumin, garlic, lemongrass, onion, pepper, salt
Oriental Seasoning	

Tropical & Exotic Fruits

Acerola (usually in powdered form)	tropical, cranberry-size bright red fruit with highest vitamin C content
Asian pear	apple-like fruit with sandy-textured flesh
Dragonfruit	reddish-dark neutral-flavored oval tropical fruit with "petals", used in juices
Feijoa	sweet oval green tropical fruit, slightly smaller than kiwifruit, thick skin
Goji berry	Asian/Himalayan raisin-sized oval ruby-colored "superfood" berry,
Guava	musky/pungent-flavored green fruit; remove skin, slice & eat.
Kiwifruit	fuzzy brown fruit with succulent sweet green flesh, small edible seeds. Peel skin
Kumquat	small orange 1.5" oval citrus fruit, with a bittersweet taste, eaten whole
Lychee	Asian fruit, often used for bright yellow refreshing juice
Mandarin orange	popular, sweet mini-orange, used in salads and to garnish stir-fries, etc.
Mango	5 inch red-orange-green fruit with large seed & yellow flesh. Peel & eat raw
Mangosteen	"superfruit" with large white pit. Used often in juices.
Noni	greenish fruit usually from Tahiti known for bitter taste but great health benefits
Papaya (Carica papaya)	pear-shaped fruit with peppery seeds. Highly digestive if skin & flesh are green
Passionfruit	purplish fruit that is wrinkly when ripe, pale green succulent flesh inside
Pepino melon	edible yellow green-striped skin. Apple & honeydew melon taste, crisp as plum
Pineapple	spiny skin, sweet yellow flesh good for digestion(bromelain), healing skin rash
Quince	eat cooked(baked apple-pear taste). Bitter starch taste when raw.
Star Fruit (a.k.a. carambola?)	fruit with star-shaped profile, refreshing pale flesh with edible skin
Tamarillo	kiwi-sized dark-red edible fruit with smooth skin, of Nightshade family.
Cherimoya	decadent creamy-fleshed fruit, French-white-sauce texture. Remove seeds, skin

Kitchen Safety & Good Practice

Spills (salt reduces slippage)	Fingers are valuable! Use care with knives, mixer, blender, grater, mandoline!
Chemicals	Clean up immediately, **especially** oil(slipping on oil=dangerous & painful!)
Labeling (throw out after 6 days)	must be separated from food/food contact surfaces, in original containers
Cleaning knives	Labeled with food name and date(month & make-day) when put in cold storage
	Clean after use with cloth, brush/sponge & soapy water. Air dry on clean surface

Equipment & Utensils Needed

	ITEM
appliances	Bread machine
	can opener
	refrigerator
	food processor and/or nut grinder
	fry pan/skillet, griddle or flat top grill (pancakes)
	mixer--5-quart- with paddle, whisk, and dough hook
	pressure cooker or rice cooker
	stove/burners, oven
	Vitamix or blender, food processor if possible
	work table
bowls	mixing bowls: 2-gallon,1-gallon,2-quart, 1-quart,1 pint--stainless steel(pref.)
	salsa bowls (3-6 inches across)
food prep	cherry pitter, paring knife, or fingers!
	coffeemaker w/filters
	cutting board:12x18 to 18x24
	graters-large hole and small hole (fine grating), zester
	9"-18" colander/strainer
	melon-baller--3/4" (double), lemon juicer
	mortar & pestle
	spritzer
	sprouter, either "Sproutamo" or Mason jar with screened lid
	teapot
	vegetable slicer (mandoline, etc.)
general	clean kitchen towels for covering flour while raising
	faucet with hot & cold running water with at least 2 sinks
	paper towels
	plates or saucers for rolling balls in coatings
	wax paper
handling	oven mitts and thermometer, timer
measuring	measuring cups: 1/8,1/4,1/3,1/2,1--stainless steel, or plastic--two of each
	measuring cups--large: 1 cup,2 cup, 4 cup/1 quart, 2 quart, 1 gallon X
	measuring spoons
	gram-ounce-pound scale (digital even better but not necessary)
	baker/dough scale
pans	baking pans with 1/2"-1" rims
	breadpans -- 9x5x4"
	cake pans (regular, Bundt) and muffin pans, pie pans, wire cooling racks
	cookie sheets
	12"-15" pizza pan, sauce pan, frying pan or wok, soup pot (6-8 quart)
pantry	well-stocked (and fresh) herb and spice shelf/pantry
serving	casserole dish--9x13x2 inch and 8x8x2
	lasagna pan
	parfait glasses and/or pudding dishes
	serving platter
utensils	12"-18" kitchen spoons: wooden, stainless steel, pizza cutter, pastry brush
	salad tongs, knives(chef, paring, bread), metal spatulas, rolling pin, flour sifter
	1"-3" teaball, cake spatulas, rubber spatulas, whisk
	toothpicks for checking cakes
	vegetable scrubbing brush, vegetable peeler
	TOTAL

Aminos, Brain, Healing, Enzymes

X = supplied by Bragg Liquid Aminos
Recommended:

Amino Acids, essential [7]	**Essential amino acids not made by body, must be supplied by diet.** [7]
Histidine X	tissue growth/repair, myelin sheath, red & white blood cells, heavy metal removal
Isoleucine X	hemoglobin, stabilize blood sugar/energy level,energy,endurance,muscle repair
Leucine X	protect muscle, fuel,heal bone/skin/muscle, blood-sugar balance, growth hormones
Lysine X	protein builder,growth,nitrogen balance,collagen,lower triglycerides,fight herpes virus
Methionine X	fat breakdown,digestive health,de-tox heavy metals,strengthen muscle,osteoporosis
Phenylalanine X	raise mood,reduce pain,memory/learning, arthritis,depression, obesity, brain health
Threonine X	protein balance,collagen/elastin formation,liver function/prevent fat buildup,antibodies
Tryptophan	Niacin & serotonin source, normal sleep, anti-stress, growth hormone release
Valine X	stimulant effect,muscle metabolism,tissue repair,nitrogen balance,muscle energy

Amino Acids, non-essential [7]

Alanine X	glucose metabolism,constituent of pantothenic acid(B5)
Arginine X	enhances immune function, T cells,sexual maturity,healing tissue,muscles,nitrogen
Asparagine	balance of central nervous system,amino acid transformation
Aspartic Acid X	increase stamina,neural & brain health,ammonia removal,blood detoxifier,RNA/DNA
Cysteine,Cystine(sister aminos)	skin,detoxifier,nails/skin/hair health,collagen,surgical healing,chelates heavy metals
Dimethylglycine(from Glycine)	Energy, mental acuity, immunity enhancer, reduce cholesterol, oxygenation
Gamma Aminobutyric Acid	neurotransmitter,brain metabolism/function,calm nerve cells, regulate sex hormones
Glutamic Acid(neurotransmitter) X	increase neuron firing,sugar/fat metabolism,detoxify ammonia,personality disorders
Glutamine	brain fuel,acid/alkaline balance,RNA/DNA synthesis,mental ability,digestion, health
Glutathione (tripeptide)	powerful antioxidant,blood cell integrity,carbohydrate metabolism, fat breakdown
Glycine X	retard muscle degeneration,nucleic acid synthesis,bile acid, repair damaged tissues
Proline X	skin collagen production,health of connective tissue,joints & heart muscle
Serine X	fatty acid metabolism,muscle growth,immunity,immunoglobulin,antibody,moisturizer
Taurine	amino building block,fat digestion,mineral utilization,restore potassium,protect brain
Tyrosine X	norepinephrine/dopamine precursor,regulate mood,reduce body fat,endocrine glands

Brain Foods [7]

Lecithin (granules or liquid)	human cell need,myelin sheath,anti-arteriosclerosis,improve brain function,energy
Choline	component of lecithin, B-vitamin,necessary for nerve transmission impulses,memory
Inositol	component of lecithin, B-vitamin, promotes emotional stability
Omega 3 Essential Fatty Acids	alpha-linolenic, eicosapentaenoic acid:canola, flaxseed, walnut
Omega 6 Essential Fatty Acids	linoleic,gamma-linolenic:nuts,seeds,peanut,borage,grape seed,primrose,sesame,soy
Gotu Kola	decrease fatigue/depression, central nervous system stimulant, good for circulation
Ginkgo biloba	blood circulation, oxygenate heart,brain,body,improve memory,ear health,impotence
Kelp	eat raw or dry.salt substitute.B vitamins,iodine.Benefits brain,nerves,obesity(thyroid)
Folic Acid	B-vitamin, prevents neural-tube defects (fetal development of new-born baby)

Blood--cleanse, build, heal [7]

red clover	used for "spring cleanses", known to have anti-cancer effects,nitrogen-fixing
chlorophyll	internal deodorant,nutrient-rich,plentiful in parsley,alfalfa,chlorella, green vegetables
beet root	flavorful bright red root, used as vegetable, raw (grated) or cooked, good blood-builder
beet greens	must be cooked or steamed to "sit well" on the digestive system.
alfalfa	chlorophyll-rich,minerals,nutrients,absorbs well; ulcers,eczema,liver,anemia,infection
shiitake mushroom	T cell booster,18 amino acids,rich in B1,B2,B3,effective for cancer,entirely edible
reishi mushroom	youth, longevity,superior medicine,prevent high blood pressure,edible
Maitake mushroom	Well-absorbed mushroom,edible,adaptogen,inhibit cancer & HIV,boost T-helper cells

Enzymes 101   hint: good reason to eat raw plant-based foods!
Unchanging proteins in the body that help chemical reactions occur, but do not get used up themselves
Some 2000 enzymes speed the rate of chemical & metabolic reactions by a factor from 10 up to a million-plus.

Aminos, Brain, Healing, Enzymes

Specific enzymes must be available in order for reactions in the body to occur fast enough.
Are killed by heat exceeding 112 degrees Fahrenheit (44 degrees Celsius)

BRAIN DRAINERS	Description	Found in/sources/causes:
Mercury	toxic metal	vaccines, agricultural chemicals, coal product, dental work
Lead	toxic metal	solder, adhesive for stained glass windows, old paint
Excess Vitamin A	animal source	conventional supplements
Nicotine	nerve toxin	found in tobacco products
Alcohol	ethyl alcohol	cleaner/fermented beverage
Stress		typical human situation in varying degrees
Sedentary (lazy) lifestyle		habitual TV watching, laying around, processed high-fat/low-nutrient foods
Obesity		more than 30 pounds over ideal weight, primarily fat weight
	overfed & undernourished	food choices, hypo-metabolism
		taking in more calories (typically empty calories) than are burned by metabolism or exercise

Omegas 3 & 6; HDL, LDL

Essential Fatty Acids	Comments
Omega 3 [7]	double bond occurs between the 3rd and 4th carbons from the CH3 end(Omega)
Omega 3 functions:	structure & function of cell membranes, retina of eye, and central nervous system
1) alpha-linolenic acid	vegetable oils, including canola and soybean oils
2) eicosapentaenoic acid	polyunsaturated oil, involved in cellular activity
3) docosahexanoic acid	fish oils (tuna, salmon, etc.)
4) Arachidonic Acid	works with DHA(docosahexanoic acid) to provide brain development in children
canola oil	from flower grown specifically for its oil; remains liquid in refrigeration
flaxseed oil	Flax (Linum usitatissimum)---brown and golden seeds, both are similar in benefit
walnut oil	typically Juglans regia[English walnut]

Omega 6 [7] Acids	1st double bond occurs between 6th & 7th carbon from Omega end
Omega 6 functions:	growth, red blood cell structure, skin integrity, fertility
1) linoleic acid	$C_{18}H_{32}O_2$, typically found in peanut oil, corn, sunflower, soybean & safflower oils
2) gamma-linolenic	$C_{18}H_{30}O_2$, found in flax oil, essential for wellness.
raw nuts	(almond, walnut, hazelnut, pistachio, Brazil, pecan, macadamia, etc.)
seeds	(sunflower, pumpkin, sesame, chia, etc.)
oil-releasing legumes	soybean, peanuts, etc.)
borage oil	oil from borage (borago officinalis) plant
grape seed oil	somewhat bitter oil, from winemaking process
primrose oil	Evening Primrose, enhances both testosterone and estrogen release
sesame oil	EFA content difference in untoasted vs. toasted oil unknown, or trivial
soybean oil	poly-unsaturated oil with neutral flavor used in salad dressings, frying oil, etc.
Trans-fatty Acid	hydrogens are on opposite sides of double bond (trans configuration), high melting point
Benefits of EFA's:	improvement of skin and hair, lowered blood pressure, arthritis prevention,
	brain development and function, learning & memory recall,
	prevention of candidiasis, cardiovascular diseases, eczema, and psoriasis

***Heat destroys the essential fatty acids

Daily requirement of EFA's is 10-20% of total caloric intake
    Ex: on 2000-calorie diet, 200-400 calories to be EFA's

Unsaturated Fats:	kinks and bends in molecules prevent them from fitting closely; vegetable source, melt at cooler temperatures, bound to only 1 hydrogen
Mono-unsaturated:	most common: oleic acid (olive & canola); 1 double bond in the molecule's carbon chain
Poly-unsaturated:	most common: linoleic acid (corn, safflower, soybean), more than 1 double bond
Saturated Fats:	non-kinking=[more sticking together]=solid masses at high temperature; each carbon has 2 hydrogens bound to it ("saturated" with hydrogen), no carbon-carbon double bonds
	most common: palmitic acid (16 carbons): vegetable sources: palm oil, palm kernel oil, coconut oil
	stearic acid (primarily animal products), 18 carbons
Cholesterol 101	**FACT: human body makes its own cholesterol; no cholesterol in vegetable oils**
HDL=High Density Lipoprotein: (good)	high protein:lipid ratio, carry good cholesterol to liver for elimination
	High HDL=low risk of heart disease; HDL raised by exercise
	HDL lowered by cigarette smoking
LDL=Low Density Lipoprotein: (bad)	high lipid:protein ratio, carry cholesterol to cells and blood vessels
	athero= artery, sclerosis=hardening, or stiff & unflexible arteries

Produce

Produce with ROY G. BIV — **Green is our middle name!**
Garden, field, orchard & vineyard — With so much variety, how could "vegan" ever be boring??

RED Foods

acerola cherry	tropical fruit rich in vitamin C, usually in powdered form
cherry	several varieties: Bing, Montmorency, black (think Black Forest Cake),
cranberry	tart berry, red=ripe, raw or cooked, juice, jello, salad, vitamin C, balance H. pylori
dulse seaweed	dark red-brown, seaweed/bacon taste. Rich in iodine=good for thyroid=weight
grapefruit	sour citrus fruit, white & red flesh varieties, juice refreshing when dizzy or tired
peppers, bell	non-spicy peppers that are red, yellow, etc., when ripened/mature
peppers, chili	Anaheim, cayenne, habanero, jalapeno, peperoncini, poblano, serrano, shishito, etc.
pomegranate	Mediterranean "superfruit" --seeds are edible, skin & white "pith" are not edible
raspberry	delicious, "slimming" berry, syrups, vinaigrettes, add to green tea, desserts, etc.
red clover	flower with pinkish oval head known for its medicinal properties
Red Flame grapes	good table/snacking grapes
red onions	used for salads and as fresh vegetable garnish, pizza, sauteed vegetables, etc.
red radish	refreshing, zesty but not spicy, used in salads
red tomatoes	used in salsa, pizza, soup, salads, dressings/sauces, sandwiches, etc.
rosehips	rosebud "fruit" (dog rose[Rosa canina]), rich in Vitamin C, pleasant flavor
strawberry	the heart-shaped fruit, good with chocolate, in ice cream, on fruit pizza, etc.
Thompson grapes	table grapes
watermelon	refreshing snack on hot day, best eaten alone or with other melons, hydrating
lettuce, Red Leaf	used often in lettuce mixes such as spring mix or other salads

ORANGE Foods

acorn squash (winter)	bake, add molasses, brown sugar & cinnamon, use as edible bowl. Roast seeds
apricot	desserts, breads, jam/jelly, eat fresh, high beta carotene & copper, good for acne
butternut squash (winter)	delicious squash, great in minestrone, as its own soup, or vegetable/grain dish
cantaloupe	delicious, popular orange, refreshing melon to eat by itself (high water content)
carrots	rabbits don't wear glasses! High beta carotene. salad, soup, casseroles, juice
Hubbard squash (winter)	saw in half (squash is at least 12" in diameter), then place in oven
kumquat	small bitter-sweet oval citrus fruit the size of a large olive.
mandarin oranges	famous tangerine-like fruit in Asian foods (Mandarin is main language in China)
orange	versatile fruit--desserts, baked goods, snack, smoothies, spice cake, vitamin C
papaya	digestive(papain), green skin(white flesh)=most papain, ripe=soft reddish flesh
peppers, orange	Bell, habanero, etc.
pumpkin	autumn harvest, decorating, pumpkin pie, raw inside flesh is bitter
red lentils	much-used Indian food("Dal"), small but bright-colored, high in iron, protein
sweet potato	high beta-carotene, satisfying, sweet, great with fruit, grains, vegetables
tangerine	sweet and delicious member of citrus family, used for juices, desserts, snacks

Produce

YELLOW Foods

bamboo	feeds panda bears, fastest growing grass, most edible grass, light flavor
calendula (marigold officinalis)	called "pot marigold". yes, you can eat the petals! And they are good for healing
casaba melon	another refreshing melon, available in autumn, typically yellow flesh
corn	salsa, chowder, flour, chips, corn-on-the-cob, tortilla soup, polenta, etc.
crenshaw melon	another under-used refreshing cool-season melon
ginger	widely-used rhizome spice, Asian, Creole, Indian, good with fruit, vegetables, breads, etc.
gold flax seed	Omega-3, reportedly has more Omega 3 than brown flax, same uses
lemon	yellow, pungent & somewhat astringent citrus fruit
lettuce, Belgian Endive	say "Ahn-DEEV", (French) oval yellow-green lettuce
mango	juicy, rich in vitamin A and C, texture a bit slippery, unique peachy taste, large seed
millet (grain)	Rich in Vitamin B, powerhouse grain, gluten-free cous-cous, use with rice, etc.
muskmelon	yellowish-green inside flesh
nectarine	the sweeter "cousin" of peaches, with no hair.
olive oil	the more virgin the oil, the yellower the color, the more pungent-fruity the flavor
peach	famous for pies and snacks, both red-orange flesh and white flesh varieties
pine nuts (a.k.a. pinoli)	from Italian Stone Pine, Mediterranean; dolmas, dessert, salads, parmesan taste
pineapple	pina colada, smoothies, banana splits, digestion (bromelain), heals skin rashes
spaghetti squash	flesh has spaghetti-like fibers after cooking, delicious gluten-free spaghetti meal
summer squash, Chayote	
summer squash, Pattypan	looks like a squashed mini-pumpkin
summer squash, yellow crookneck	salads, soups, casseroles, steamed vegetables
yam (use without skin)	white, yellow or creamy flesh color, best cooked
yellow onion	used mostly for cooking, mild flavor
yellow peppers	banana, caribe, bell, wax
yellow split pea	mostly used in Indian foods, or pilafs
yellow tomatoes	use like red tomatoes
Yukon Gold potatoes	gold-colored creamy flesh, more flavor, add color to ordinary dishes, soup, etc.

Produce

GREEN Foods

alfalfa	blood purifier, freshening, use sprouts on sandwiches, salads, herb in tea, food
artichoke, globe	artichoke most often used in Italian & Mediterranean cooking.
asparagus	used mainly as side dishes, or with pasta primavera, etc.
avocados	creamy-fleshed fruit of Mexican fame; garnish, guacamole, salsa/sauce, healthy fats & protein
beet greens	Another family of greens that should be cooked, very cleansing properties
Bok Choy	Chinese cabbage like Nappa, but with much darker leaf, more pungent stem
broccoli	green version of cauliflower, steam large pieces, use small pieces raw, with dip
broccoli raab, broccolini	broccoli hybrids
brussels sprouts	bite-size cabbages from Belgium. Usually cooked
celeriac (Apiaceae graveolens)	celery plant with large tap root. Slice off outer skin of root, use raw or cooked
celery	in French "mire poix" (carrots, celery, onions). Soups, eat raw, & with nut butters
collards	"Southern greens", usually cooked
cucumber	long dark green cooling summer vegetable, often used for pickles
dandelion leaf	Those annoying weeds in your yard can actually benefit your kidneys
fava beans	Middle Eastern/Mediterranean. Used in baking flour, steamed, falafel, etc. Cook & peel beans
feijoa (tropical fruit)	say "fay-hoh-a". Kiwifruit-sized with large garlic-shaped pit inside. Only inside flesh is edible
fennel	Celery-like stalks from a bulb. Delicious leaves, stalk tastes like licorice
French green lentils	dark "marbled" green lentils with earthy flavor
green beans	thin version "haricot vert(French--areekoh vair)", or Italian beans, wide and flat
green cabbage	used raw for coleslaw, or cooked in stuffed cabbage, soups, sauerkraut, etc.
green grapes	refreshing, light-tasting grape used with both fruits and vegetable salads
green onions (a.k.a. scallions)	compact onion taste, good as garnish. Often used with Mexican foods, potato salad, etc.
green peppers	technically not ripe at this stage, but chockfull of vitamin C!
guava (tropical fruit)	thick-skinned fruit, kiwifruit-sized. Inside flesh edible, can be made into juice. several varieties
honeydew melon	beige skin, refreshing green flesh, typically available in summer
kale	Blue (blue-green), Scotch, and Lacinato(longer, slender leaf) varieties available
kelp seaweed	brown leaves, greenish powder. Unique "lake" taste. Rich in iodine (metabolism-boost)
kiwi fruit	sweet green flesh with small edible seeds. Scoop out flesh to eat
leek	very large, thick green onion, mild-tasting, used in soups & casseroles, etc.
lemon grass	lemony-tasting grass, grown as long, woody stalks, use tender part of stalk
lettuce, arugula (rocket)	say "a-ROO-gula", peppery taste, high in Vitamin C, often used in spring mix
lettuce, Boston/Bibb lettuce	sandwiches, bed of lettuce
lettuce, buttercup	sandwiches, bed of lettuce
lettuce, curly leaf Endive	mesclun, other various uses
lettuce, escarole	say "ES-ka-roll", a bit bitter, usually in spring mix, frilly leaves add "gourmet touch"
lettuce, loose leaf	lettuce used mostly for sandwiches(lays flat)
lettuce, romaine	principally used in Caesar salad, various other uses
lime	three types: standard lime (~ 2 1/2" long), Key Lime (~ 1 1/4" long) & Kaffir lime (Thai, Indian)
mesclun (early spring greens)	mix of young greens such as spinach, arugula, chicory, radicchio, frisee, escarole, etc.
mustard greens	narrow 8" leaves with slightly spicy mustard-radish taste, flat leaf & curly leaf varieties
Napa (Chinese) cabbage	oval-shaped cabbage with lots of pale green leaves and pleasant mild taste
okra	mucilaginous skinny pepper-shaped vegetable famous in Cajun gumbo, breaded, fried, raw
peas	garden peas, split peas, sugar snap peas(thick, round), snow peas (thin, wide)
pistachio	delightful-tasting green nut with Mediterranean origin, use in pudding, eat raw, etc.
pumpkin seeds	(without the white husk), rich in zinc, earthy flavor
rhubarb	long green/red stalk cooked or eaten raw. Leaves and roots are toxic
savoy cabbage	dark green veiny round cabbage, used in soups such as minestrone, or salad, etc.
spinach	dark green iron-rich leaf good in salads, casseroles, pasta, smoothies, spanakopita(Greek pie)
sprouts	rich in nutrients, the only problem is waiting the 3-5 days for them to sprout!
Swiss Chard	rich, green flavor, delicious cooked or steamed, leaves and stems edible
tomatillo	Mexico's "green tomato", mild taste, just peel off the outer husk, cut and eat.
turnip greens	young leaves can be used raw (mesclun, salads), mature leaves must be cooked
ugli fruit	big, round, green citrus fruit with refreshing taste, bumpy version of pommelo
watercress	small-leafed salad green or garnish
zucchini	long dark green summer squash used in relishes, salads, casseroles, stir-fries

Produce

Blue/Dark Red/Purple Foods

acai fruit	say "ah-sigh-ee", small purple "superfruit" from Brazil, used in juices,healing
beet	probably the healthiest root vegetable, use raw or cooked, salads,with grains;(greens edible)
bilberry	slightly smaller, European version of blueberry
black raspberry	
blackberry	
blue corn flour	used by the Hopi Indians for stamina, different but good taste,good as chips
blue potatoes	unique taste, but good and fairly creamy taste
blueberry	round blue totally edible berry, good in salads, fruit pizza, pies, smoothies, cobblers, etc.
boysenberry	dark purple version of raspberry, a bit bigger
Concord grapes	dark purple table grapes, often used in red wine, juice, jams/jellies
eggplant	pear-shaped purple vegetable with fat-absorbing qualities.Ratatouille,moussaka,
elderberry	reputed medicinal berry, must cook before eating/drinking.Good for flu,colds
Emperor's Purple Rice	dark purple rice,originally forbidden for use by any other than the Emperor
logan berry 4	hybrid of blackberry & red raspberry
marion berry	similar to black raspberry
mulberry	small, purple, cylindrical berry coming from tall trees. Snacks,cereal,etc.
passion fruit	wrinkled = ripe. scoop out juicy flesh and seeds; has citrusy-bitter peach flavor
plum	red plums & black plums
prune	dried plum, high iron content, used for increasing dietary fiber
radicchio lettuce	say "ra-DEE-keeo", dark red and white cabbage/lettuce, used often in mesclun
red cabbage	purple cabbage used in coleslaw, soups, etc.

OTHER (brown, white, etc.) Foods

almond	seed of an apricot-like fruit, mass produced for its healthy qualities and oil
aloe vera	soothing and healing for the inside and the outside of the body, natural laxative
amaranth (Incan supergrain)	excellent source of iron, very small grain, can also use for sprouting
apples	abundant & popular American fruit, healthy skin & flesh, toxic seeds(cyanide)
arborio rice (used in risotto)	short grain rice used in Italy for rice dishes, both white and brown varieties
Asian pear	gritty textured white flesh, apple-pear taste
banana (Cavendish)	yellow-skinned long slender fruit with white dry flesh. Ripe fruit good in baking
beans	adzuki,anasazi,black,canellini,soy,garbanzo,kidney,mung,red,pinto,borlotti,fava
black japonica rice	black variety of rice, found in Old World Pilaf,supposedly cultivated in Japan
Brazil nut	large nut highest in mineral Selenium.
brown flaxseed	brown version, same uses and similar benefits as gold flax
brown rice	easily-digestible gluten-free grain used by many cultures
buckwheat	gluten-free grain, green-brown color, pointed on one end,"Kashi"~ in Europe
burdock root	liver support, needs to be cooked (either tea or use root as a vegetable)
cacao (Theobroma cacao)	(cocoa bean). Plant origin of chocolate.
cashew	fatty nut with complex shelling process, Asian & Indian foods,cream,snacking
cauliflower	cabbage-family, looks like a thundercloud, bland, crunchy; soup,salad,good steamed
chayote squash(Sechium edule) 2	green or white fruits eaten cooked, boiled or raw. Young roots are cooked like potatoes
chestnuts	Olde English nut, apparently good roasted. Christmas song named after it
chia seeds	South American/Latin American "energy" food. Seeds make gel when soaked
coconut	large tropical nut used for milk, juice, flakes/shredding, oil, desserts, snacking
currant (Ribes nigrum 'Consort')	zante currant, small berry, often dried, use for jellies & sauce, cereal, snacking
Daikon radish	large, mild, a bit zesty, beige-colored radish; scrub well, process like a carrot
dates	Medjool, Deglet-noor... remove seed.Natural energy.Add figs to cleanse colon
figs	mission,Turkish,often dried. whole fruit is edible (remove stem), good flavor, high in calcium
filberts/hazelnuts	same nut, different names, rich in Vitamin E,good flavor,roasted for cappucino & desserts
garlic	King of herbs, with sulfur content & famous aroma. Anti-bacterial/viral/cancer…
horseradish	radish with a definite "bite"; 1/2" square clears your sinus. Use in sushi, cocktail sauce,dips
Jerusalem artichoke	different from Globe artichoke, actually a tuber(root-like), good for diabetes
jicama	similar to turnip, larger, with a bit more zest. Pico de gallo, "Mexican potato", eat raw or cooked
kohlrabi	looks like tendrils rising from the root. Member of the cabbage family.
macadamia nut	creamy nut mostly from Hawaii, and other tropical zones. Butters,oils,snacking
mushrooms (all)	button(common),enoki,crimini,shiitake,Portabello,morel,oyster,porcini,maitake,etc.

Produce

Other (brown, white, etc.) Foods, continued

lotus root	used primarily in Asian food--appearance like horseradish root
olives (I:Italy,G:Greek,P:Peru)	black(CA),Kalamata,Halkidiki(G),Cerignola,Castelvetrano(I),Beldi(Af),Ascolana(P)
onion, sweet	white, and a bit milder than the red onion. Typically used for cooking
parsnip	tan-colored waxy root with earthy,delicious flavor,cooked,or raw. Peel first.
peanuts	used worldwide, in frying oils, snacking, peanut butter, candy, salads, etc.
pear	Anjou, Red Anjou, Bartlett, Red Bartlett, Bosc, StarKrimson, Comice, Concorde
pecans	famous good-flavored southern nut used in pies, salads, desserts, rich snack
persimmon	aromatic and flavorful green/brown/orange fruit, harvested in the fall.
plantain	South American/African/Creole version of the banana, this one must be cooked or fried
potato	Russet, and red (baby/ "new", and large size. roasted, potato salad, pancakes, soup, stirfry...
psyllium	see Thickeners, gel agents, also fiber supplement(husk preferred, or seed)
quinoa ("keen-wa"),"mother grain"	complete protein, small white, black & red seeds. Sprout,cook,use as flour
radish, icicle	not-often-seen white radish, smaller than horseradish
raisins	dried version of grapes, both green and black. Green often preserved with sulfur dioxide
red bananas	tropical mini-bananas often from Ecuador or South America
sesame seed	brown & black varieties, used for salads, oils, baking, delicious milks, tahini
shallot	onion family, zesty flavor, used in cooking, usually sauces. Combination of onion and garlic.
sorghum grain	gluten-free grain, the size of coriander seeds, plain-flavor white grain or flour
soybean	tofu, miso, edamame(raw green soybean), need to be cooked/heat-processed
sunchoke	root of sunflower (Helianthus annuus), tuber like turmeric and ginger. Can use whole & raw
sunflower seed	high quality protein, great for snacking, usually hulled, often sold in shell(better form for birds)
taro	a root vegetable used often in chips
turnip	round rosy-purple and white crispy root used raw in salads, or cooked.
walnuts, English	snacking, salads, Waldorf salad, desserts, baklava, etc.
walnuts, black	expel parasites, some like the bitter flavor and eat like English walnuts. (Great furniture wood)
water chestnuts	cooling, Asian foods; remove outer husk if buying raw, crunchy/crisp, refreshing
wehani rice	savory red rice used in Old World Pilaf, Thai cuisine
wild rice	grass-rice, savory rich flavor, typically expands up to 3 times original size

Herbs & Spices

Female Maternity Cautions:
Common Culinary/Food Herb
Medicinal Herb
Tea Medicinal Herb
Medicinal Food Herb

C P/B: Do not use more than culinary quantities while breastfeeding or pregnant
P/B: Do not use while breastfeeding or pregnant
E P/B: Do not eat while breastfeeding or pregnant---topical application is safe

1 Descriptions

Herb	Description
aloe vera (Aloe barbadensis) E P/B	succulent cactus-like plant with healing properties (for skin & internal);
anise seed (Pimpinella anisum) C P/B	licorice-like flavor, baking, tea, vegetable dishes, curry, soups. Grind seeds for most flavor
arnica (Arnica montana Asteraceae) P/B	flower used for reduction of pain and swelling, used in ointments for bruised muscles,etc.
basil (Ocimum sp. Lamiaceae)	great culinary & Italian herb, many varieties, major ingredient of pesto,can deter flies,etc.
bay (Laurus nobilis Lauraceae)	soup flavoring (remove leaf before eating/serving), "Bouquet garni" herb mix, garam masala
bergamot (Monarda sp. Laminaceae) P/B	use leaves for digestive complaints,fever. Not equivalent to bergamot essential oil
borage (Borago officinalis) P/B	seed oil used, rich in GLA Omega-6 oils, leaves used for skin health & swelling as a poultice
burdock root (Arctium lappa) P/B	brownish-white root used for liver support & health, purify blood,cooking:raw or in stir-fries
calendula (marigold) (C. officinalis) E P/B	edible flower petals, coloring, garnish, skin-healing properties,
caraway (Carum carvi) C P/B	aromatic seed. Digestive tonic, baking, meats,fruits, vegetable dishes.Leaves in salad,soup
carob, flour	from carob tree, cocoa alternative, high-calcium, low/no caffeine, good flavor
celery (Apium graveolens) C P/B (seeds)	leaf & stem used in cooking. seed is diuretic,eliminate toxins,use in soup,relish,bread,sauces
chamomile (Matricaria recutita) C P/B	flowers used. Relaxing herb (bedtime tea), pleasant flavor, heals wounds
chervil (Anthriscus cerefolium)	whole plant. French herb in "Fines Herbes" , "Herbes de Provence", like tarragon & parsley.
chickweed	all parts. Reduce mucus in lungs,bronchitis,circulatory,colds,coughs,skin disease,warts
chili peppers (Capsicum sp. Solanacaea)	green is unripe. jalapeno,habanero,bell,tabasco,cayenne,paprika,poblano,Thai,Szechuan~~
chicory	leaves, roots, roots can be brewed as caffeine-free substitute for coffee
chives (Allium schoenoprasum)	green herb similar to green onion,good with potatoes,sauces,salad dressings.heat-sensitive
coriander,cilantro (Coriandrum sativum)	leaves(like parsley),stems,seeds used in salads,soup, curry,stir-fry.Asian,Mid-East,Mexican
comfrey (Symphytum officinale) P/B	use leaves & roots.healing to skin(**do not eat**), use only externally as poultice or in ointment
curry plant (Helichrysum italicum)	fresh leaves & stems(sprigs) used to flavor foods with "curry" flavor
dandelion (Taraxacum officinale) C P/B	leaves as salad greens, kidney health,root used for liver,digestive support,coffee substitute
damiana	hormonal tonic,intestinal contractions,oxygenate genitals,aphrodisiac,female sexual tonic
dill (Anethum graveolens) C P/B	use leaves on salads,soup,vegetables,potatoes, seeds in pickles,bread(rye),digestive tonic
dong quai (Angelica archangelica)	roots are used,digestive tonic,hormone support, "barbeque" flavor,young shoots in salads
Echinacea (purpurea,angustifolia) P/B	roots,leaves,flowers and seed used.immune support,cold/flu,respiratory,infections
elder (Sambucus nigra) P/B	flowers & berries used. Cold,flu,mucus reduction,immune support. berries must be cooked.
eucalyptus (Corymbia sp.Myrtaceae) P/B	leaf oils are repellent to most insects,has antibacterial/antiviral properties, decongestant
Evening Primrose (Oenothera) P/B	seed oil used, high in GLA Omega 6, anti-inflammatory, best when taken with Omega-3
Eyebright (Euphrasia officinalis) P/B	leaves,flowers used.Nasal secretions,congestion,eye health,hay fever,compress for eyes
Fennel (Foeniculum vulgare) C P/B	Leaves:salads;root:vegetable;seed:food flavor,digestive aid,increase breast milk,respiratory
fenugreek (Trigonella foenum-graecum)	sinus/mucus problems, blood sugar, cholesterol, delicious soothing tea,add to cooking food
Flax (Linum usitatissimum) P/B	seed used for food,dietary fiber, Omega 3-rich,egg-replacer,linseed oil,flax oil,baking,cereal
Galangal (Alpinia galanga) C P/B	not as strong as ginger. Indian/Asian foods,sambals,ras el hanout.digestive tonic
Garlic (Allium sativum) C P/B	anti-microbial,anti-cancer, heart health. soups,vegetables,bake in foil for a spread,
Ginger root (Zingiber officinale)	digestive tonic, colds, warming, arthritis, cardiovascular.Use in stews,curry,salad,chutney
Ginkgo biloba P/B	leaves,fruit.Brain health,enhance blood flow,anti-inflammatory,protect cells.Autumn harvest
Ginseng (Panax, Eleuteroccus) P/B	energizing herb,adaptogen(stress),mental function,endurance,blood sugar
Gotu kola (Centella asiatica) P/B	whole plant,leaves used. Skin rejuvenation,nerve & brain health,longevity,vein health
golden seal(alcohol-free extract best form)	immune support,antibiotic,cleanse body,anti-inflammatory,insulin catalyst,gland function
hibiscus (Hibiscus sabdariffa)	red calyces(surrounding base of yellow flowers)used for making sauce,jelly,cool drinks,tea
hyssop (Hyssopus officinalis) P/B	stem,leaf,flower.respiratory/lung health,antibacterial/viral,colds,flu,calming,herpes sores
jasmine (Jasminum)	flowers,roots.Essential oil used for skin problems,antidepressant,relaxant.Flavor for tea,rice
lavender (Lavandula officinalis)	flowers. Antiseptic, antibacterial,blemished skin, moth-repellent,relieve anxiety,restful sleep
lemon balm (Melissa officinalis) P/B	leaves have lemon-mint flavor,use for tea,fruit,salads and stuffing;sedative,enhances mood
lemon grass (Cymbopogon citratus) C P/B	used mostly in Asian food or in tea, oil is insect repellent,digestive tonic,pain relief

Herbs & Spices

lemon verbena (Aloysia citriodora) P/B	leaves used sparingly in teas, salads,with fruit, Asian dishes.Can substitute for lemon grass
licorice root (Glycyrrhiza glabra) P/B	digestive tonic, tea, respiratory,adrenal gland tonic,used in Chinese master stocks for flavor
lime (Tilia cordata) P/B	not related to the citrus family.Also known as linden.Dried flowers used for lime blossom tea
lovage (Levisticum officinale)	leaves like celery,stems blanched or raw,seeds for breads,pastries.Aphrodisiac,deodorant
marjoram (Origanum) C P/B	herb milder than oregano,heat damages aroma;essential oil:pain,digestive,respiratory
meadowsweet (Filipendula ulmaria) P/B	flowers,leaves.Digestive tonic,balance stomach acid,aspirin-like properties.Jams & fruits
mint (Mentha) C P/B, oil: P/B	peppermint,spearmint,etc.Leaves for digestive discomfort,use in yogurt,jelly,lamb,salads,tea
milk thistle (leaves, seeds)	liver support
oregano (Origanum vulgare) C P/B	Leaves. Italian, Mexican, Greek varieties,etc. colds,fever,digestive tonic,antimicrobial
parsley (Petroselinum) C P/B	leaves,roots,seeds.Herb mixes,digestive tonic,chlorophyll, breath freshener,diuretic,curative
passionflower (Passiflora incarnata) P/B	flower used for anxiety & stress; fruits from P. edulis (passionfruit),inside flesh eaten
perilla (Perilla fruitescens) C P/B	Asian herb.red variety for food.Leaves:color & flavor pickled foods,sprout seeds for salads
plantain (Plantago) P/B	psyllium from P. psyllium (husk & seed a good fiber source), P.lanceolata, anti-inflammatory
poppy (Papaver rhoeas,Escholzia california) P/B	seed used for baked goods, breads, pastries, etc.
red clover (Trifolium pratense) P/B	flowers,young leaves used for blood-cleansing, delicious tea,skin & respiratory,menopause
rocket/arugula (Eruca sativa)	leaves:lettuce with peppery flavor. Salads,pizza,risotto,soups.Sprout seeds.High in C & iron
rosehips,petals (Rosa canina,gallica) C P/B	vitamin C,makes delicious syrup,rosewater(Turkish Delight),petals of R. gallica "Officinalis"
rosemary (Rosmarinus officinalis)	popular aromatic herb,pungent pine-like flavor, nerve tonic,circulation,memory,concentration
St. John's Wort (Hypericum perforatum)P/B	flowering tops. Nerve pain, anxiety & depression
saffron (Crocus sativus) P/B	stigmas from crocuses. Used for yellow/orange/red coloring. Used in rice, vegetables, etc.
sage (Salvia officinalis(culinary))	leaves."Thanksgiving dinner" herb,anti-inflammatory/microbial,use with beans,soups,stuffing
savory (Satureja hortensis & montana)	summer,winter savory leaves. Lentils,soups,sauces,Herbes de Provence
sarsaparilla	energizing herb (root),increase energy,regulates hormones,protects against radiation
sassafras	leaf used in Cajun gumbo file (herbal seasoning blend)
slippery elm	Inner bark used. Soothes inflamed mucous membranes. Used for diarrhea,ulcers,colds.
sorrel(Rumex acetosa,scutatus,acetosella)	vitamin C,tangy,best when young & tender.No aluminum or iron pots(leaves turn black)
Sweet Cicely (Myrrhis odorata)	roots--tonic,boil as vegetable,stems used in salads.Leaves--anise aroma, safe for diabetics
star anise (Illicium verum) (see Anise)	pod(star) used, 5-spice powder,Chinese cooking,more aromatic/pungent than anise seed
Stevia (rebaudiana)	leaf is used as is for natural herbal sweetener
tarragon (Artemisia dracunculus)	leaves. French herb("Fines Herbes"), piquant flavor,use in dressings,mustard,sauces
thyme (Thymus vulgaris)	leaves.casseroles,marinades,jambalaya,gumbo,pates,etc. colds,expel excess mucus,
turmeric (Cucuma longa) C P/B	related to ginger. tonic,blood purifier,anti-inflammatory,digestive. Curry,chermoula,rice,lentils
valerian (Valeriana officinalis) P/B	roots used as sedative,relaxant of nervous system & muscles.
Watercress (Nasturtium officinale) P/B	high in vitamin C,peppery taste complements soups,citrus,sandwiches
White horehound (Marrubium vulgare) P/B	leaves,flowers used for bronchial conditions,colds,mucus,digestive tonic
yarrow (Achillea millefolium) P/B	leaves,stems used to heal wounds,stop bleeding,anti-inflammatory,fevers,digestive tonic
yellow dock (Rumex crispus)	related to sorrel. roots used for detoxifying liver & bowel

Trees with medicinal properties	**P/B except for topical use of witch hazel**
Magnolia (Magnolia officinalis)	bitter tonic used to improve digestion,menstrual,liver
Oak (Quercus robur)	Dried bark is astringent, anti-inflammatory,bleeding control,diarrhea,skin conditions
Walnut (Juglans nigra)	black walnut hulls used for expelling parasites & intestinal worms
Hawthorn (Crataegus)	berries used for circulatory/heart health
White willow (Salix alba)	pain-relieving, reduce swelling/inflammation
Olive (Olea europaea)	fruits (olives) used widely as food, healthy oil, leaf lowers blood pressure,anti-oxidant
Horse Chestnut (Aesculus hippocastanum)	seed provides circulatory benefits for blood vessels
Prickly Ash (Zanthoxylum americanum)	herb used for varicose veins, Raynaud's disease
Witch hazel (Hamamelis virginiana)	well-known soothing, anti-inflammatory astringent used mostly on skin,menstrual.

Herbs & Spices

Berries

Bilberry (Vaccinium myrtillus)	vision & eye health (similar to blueberry)
Saw Palmetto (Serenoa repens) P/B	healthy prostate gland (men)
Chaste Tree (Vitex agnus-castus) P/B	regulate menstrual cycle, hormonal imbalances,PMS
Cranberry (Vaccinium macrocarpon)	tart berry high in vitamin C,antioxidants,prevent cystitis(as well as H. pylori, etc.)
Schisandra (Schisandra chinensis) P/B	used for asthma,coughs,sleep disorders,liver health
Juniper (Juniperus communis) P/B	diuretic, used for gout,arthritis,rheumatism
Raspberry (Rubus idaeus)	berries are delicious, leaves used to prepare uterus for childbirth
Wild strawberry (Fragaria vesca) leaf:P/B	leaves taken to relieve mild diarrhea,minor stomach problems
Blackberry (Rubus fruticosus) leaf: P/B	berries similar to raspberry. Leaves used as strong astringent,mostly for diarrhea

Herbal energizers

Ginseng >> (see also "Herbs")	
~Siberian (Eleutherococcus senticosus)	
~Chinese/Korean (Panax ginseng)	
~American (Panax quinquefolius)	
Ashwaganda	
Astragalus (root)	immune system tonic,adrenal function,digestion,metabolism,healing,stamina, combats fatigue
Green Tea (Camellia sinensis)	antioxidant,combats mental fatigue,lower cancer risk,delays arteriosclerosis
Maca root	Peruvian origin, endurance, reproductive benefits
Muira puama	South American, male tonic, reproductive, stamina
Rhodiola rosea	Russia, Asian sources
Schisandra	Asian origin
Yerba mate	All parts used. Blood cleanser,appetite control,stimulates mind,cortisone,nerve tonic
Yohimbe	Bark used. Hormone stimulant,increases libido and blood flow to erectile tissue

Spices

allspice	Jamaican spice, a single berry that is ground up to a powder
anise seed	small aromatic seed used to flavor cookies, bread, reduce excess mucus
black pepper (Piper nigrum)	edible dried berry adding a bite to cooked vegetables,stews,etc.
capers	Mediterranean salted berry; bruschetta, Italian, Mediterranean cuisine
caraway seed	dark brown crescent-shaped aromatic rye-flavored seed; baked goods
cardamom	Indian spice, pungent aromatic green oval pods;cooking,breath freshener
celery seed	tiny brown seed used to flavor coleslaw, sauces,spice blends,etc.
cinnamon (Cinnamomum verum, C. cassia)	cider,desserts,tea,pudding, bread,Asian 5-spice powder,blood sugar health
cloves (Syzygium aromaticum)	breath freshener, "sister spice" with cinnamon,pain reliever,antiseptic,reduce swelling
coriander (cilantro seed)	Mexican, Italian, Indian foods
cumin (Cuminum cyminum)	Mexican, Italian foods, etc., reduce flatulence,colic. Added to cooking beans to reduce "gas"
fennel seed	breath freshener, many cuisines, baked goods, 5-spice powder,sausage
garlic	anti-bacterial/biotic/viral, rich in sulfur,essential body nutrient, Italian foods,etc.
ginger	Asian food, ease morning sickness, pick-me-up, digestive aid,
lemon-pepper	sweet-and-spice, variety of uses (casseroles, pasta, grains, fish, etc.)
mace (skin of nutmeg shell)	self-defense spray ingredient
mustard seed	Asian food, condiment/sauce/dressing, yellow and brown varieties,
nutmeg	eggnog, pumpkin pie spice
onion	slightly less pungent than garlic,root & stem used for food (stem called green onion, scallion)
orange peel/zest	baked goods, tea, garnishes
paprika	Slavic/Hungarian foods, coloring/flavor in chips, used in all-purpose seasonings

Herbs & Spices

Spices, continued

pepper, black	adds a bit of kick to soup, casseroles, from ripe black peppercorns
pepper, cayenne	clears sinuses effectively, very warming spice, well-known ingredient in Cajun/Creole foods
pepper, chili	Mexican, Creole, Asian foods, etc., some used for flavor, some for garnish
poppy seed	baked goods, desserts; popular in E. European/Slavic foods, lemon-poppyseed bread, etc.
saffron (Crocus sativus)	red-orange crocus pistil, gives food yellow color when cooked, use for rice, vegetables
sesame seed	Asian and Mediterranean(tahini), breads, baked goods, vegetable dip, use as milk, flavorful oil
star anise	5-spice powder, more pungent/aromatic than anise seed
tamarind (Tamarindus indica)	Mediterranean/Indian spice, also used in India as laxative, morning sickness in pregnancy
turmeric	curry powder, antibacterial, brain food, blood-clotting, dye, mustard
vanilla	long black bean-pods, baked goods, pudding, ice cream, repelling insects
Nori	sea vegetable in sheet form used to wrap sushi

Notable Healing Herbs(PNH p.64)

Cat's claw (a.k.a. Un`a de gato)	inner bark & roots. Intestinal cleanser, boost white blood cells, reduce swelling, viral infection
fig	seeds have cleansing/"scrubbing" properties, getting rid of bad bacteria, etc.
horsetail (Equisetum arvense)	rich in silica, used for skin, hair and nail health.
licorice	some aphrodisiac-like properties
milk thistle	liver health and support. best taken in capsule form.
nettle	irritant(barbed leaves), used in shampoos, herbal tinctures, etc.
pau d'arco	antibacterial, blood cleanser, candidiasis, warts, AIDS, allergies, rheumatism, tumors, ulcers
pumpkin	high beta carotene (plant source of vitamin A)
red clover	antibiotic, appetite suppressant, purify blood, relaxant, HIV, AIDS, lungs, kidney, liver, skin, immune
suma	bark, berries, leaves, roots used. For anemia, fatigue, stress, AIDS, cancer, liver, blood pressure
valerian root	sedative, use for a good night's rest, to de-stress, best in capsule form

GENERAL PRODUCE--ALL

ITEM   **(Latin names: 1)**

jasmine (Jasminum): aromatic flower used to scent rice, tea, etc.
Olive (Olea europaea): edible oil of olive (see "olive")
Evening Primrose (Oenothera) P/B (essential fatty acids)

Item	Category	Number	Codes	Notes
acai fruit	F	1	E=Energizing/adaptogenic	
acerola cherry	F	2	F=Fruit	
apples (Granny Smith, Honeycrisp, Gala, Red Delicious, etc.)	F	3	G=Grain	
apricot	F	4	H=herb	
banana (Cavendish)	F	5	I=Immune herb	
Bilberry (Vaccinium myrtillus)	F	6	S=Spice	
black raspberry	F	7	Sd=seed	
Blackberry (Rubus fruticosus) leaf:	F	8	SEA=Sea vegetable	
blueberry	F	9	Sw=sweetener	
boysenberry	F	10	V=Vegetable	
cherry	F	11		
cherimoya	F	11		
Cranberry (Vaccinium macrocarpon)	F	12		
currant (Ribes nigrum 'Consort')	F	13		
dates (Deglet-Noor, Medjool)	F	14		
dragonfruit	F	15		
feijoa (tropical fruit)	F	16		
fig-mission	F	17		
fig-Turkish/Calymyrna	F	18		
grapefruit	F	19		
grapes, Concord	F	20		
grapes, green	F	21		
grapes, Red Flame	F	22		
grapes, Thompson	F	23		
guava (tropical fruit)	F	24		
kiwi fruit	F	25		
kumquat	F	26		
lemon	F	27		
lime	F	28		
logan berry	F	29		
mandarin oranges	F	30		
mango	F	31		
marion berry	F	32		
melon, cantaloupe	F	33		
melon, casaba	F	34		
melon, Crenshaw	F	35		
melon, honeydew	F	36		
melon, kiwano	F	37		
melon, musk	F	38		
melon, pepino	F	39		
melon, watermelon	F	40		
mulberry	F	41		
nectarine	F	42		
orange (fruit, peel/zest)	F	43		
papaya	F	44		
passion fruit	F	45		
peach	F	46		
pear (Bartlett, StarKrimson, D'Anjou, Bosc, etc.)	F	47		

GENERAL PRODUCE--ALL

pear, Asian	F	48
persimmon	F	49
pineapple	F	50
plum (red, black)	F	51
pomegranate	F	52
prune	F	53
raisins	F	54
Raspberry (Rubus idaeus)	F	55
red bananas	F	56
star fruit/carambola	F	57
strawberry	F	58
tangerine	F	59
ugli fruit	F	60
amaranth (Incan supergrain)	G	1
blue corn flour	G	2
buckwheat	G	3
millet	G	4
quinoa (White,Red,Black)	G	5
rice, arborio (used in risotto)	G	6
rice, black japonica	G	7
rice, brown (short, medium and long grain)	G	8
rice, brown basmati	G	9
rice, brown jasmine	G	10
Rice, Emperor's Purple	G	11
rice, Himalayan Pink	G	12
rice, wehani	G	13
rice, wild	G	14
sorghum grain	G	15
alfalfa	H	1
aloe vera (Aloe barbadensis)	H	2
anise seed (Pimpinella anisum)	H	3
Ashwaganda	HE	4
Astragalus (root)	HE	5
basil (Ocimum sp. Lamiaceae)	H	6
bay (Laurus nobilis Lauraceae)	H	7
burdock root (Arctium lappa)	H	8
calendula (marigold officinalis)	HF	9
calendula (marigold) (C. officinalis)	H	10
caraway (Carum carvi)	H	11
Cat's claw(a.k.a. Un`a de gato)	HH	12
celery seed	H	13
Chaste Tree (Vitex agnus-castus)	H Female	14
chervil (Anthriscus cerefolium)	H	15
chives (Allium schoenoprasum)	H	16
cilantro (Coriandrum sativum)	H	17
damiana	HH	18
dandelion (Taraxacum officinale) leaf, root	H	19
dill (Anethum graveolens)	H	20
dong quai (Angelica archangelica)	HH	21
echinacea (purpurea,angustifolia)	HI	22
elderberry (Sambucus nigra)	H	23
eyebright (Euphrasia officinalis)	HM	24

GENERAL PRODUCE--ALL

Fennel (Foeniculum vulgare) seed	H	25	
fenugreek (Trigonella foenum-graecum)	H	26	
Garlic (Allium sativum) C P/B	H	27	
Ginger root (Zingiber officinale)	H	28	
ginseng: American (Panax quinquefolius)	HE	29	
ginseng: Korean (Panax ginseng)	HE	30	
ginseng: Siberian (Eleutherococcus senticosus) a.k.a. "Eleuthero"	HE	31	
golden seal(alcohol-free extract best form)	HI	32	
Gotu kola (Centella asiatica)	HE	33	
Green Tea (Camellia sinensis)	HE	34	
Hawthorn (Crataegus)	HEART	35	
hibiscus (Hibiscus sabdariffa)	HF	36	
horseradish (Brassicaceae Cruciferae)	H	37	
lavender (Lavandula officinalis)	H	38	hormonal benefits
lemon balm (Melissa officinalis)	H	39	Immunity enhancer
lemon grass (Cymbopogon citratus)	H	40	benefits prostate gland
licorice root (Glycyrrhiza glabra)	H	41	R/T=respiratory/throat
Maca root	HE	42	
marjoram (Origanum)	H	43	
milk thistle (leaves, seeds) (Sylibum)	HM	44	
mint (Mentha) oil: (peppermint,spearmint,etc.)	H	45	
Muira puama	HE	46	
oregano (Origanum vulgare)	H	47	
parsley (Petroselinum)	H	48	
pau d'arco (bark)	H	49	
psyllium	HFBR	50	S. American energizer
red clover (Trifolium pratense)	H	51	S. American energizer
Rhodiola rosea	HE	52	energizer, mental health
rosehips,petals (Rosa canina,gallica)	H	53	vitality (African origin)
rosemary (Rosmarinus officinalis)	H	54	effective energizer
saffron (Crocus sativus)	HFC	55	heart health
sage (Salvia officinalis(culinary))	H	56	use in tea, pleasant taste
sarsaparilla root	H	57	petals-food use(organic)
sassafras (Lauraceae albidum) (leaf used in Gumbo file')	H	58	fiber/laxative
savory (Satureja hortensis & montana)	H	59	food/culinary/coloring
Saw Palmetto (Serenoa repens)	H MALE	60	urinary benefits
Schisandra	HI	61	hormonal benefits
Schisandra (Schisandra chinensis)	HI	62	hormonal benefits
slippery elm	HR/T	63	Immunity enhancer
tarragon (Artemisia dracunculus)	H	64	Immunity enhancer
thyme (Thymus vulgaris)	H	65	Immunity enhancer
vanilla (bean)	H	66	eye health
yarrow (Achillea millefolium)	H	67	liver support, cleansing
yellow dock (Rumex crispus)	H	68	
Yerba mate	HE	69	
Yohimbe	HE	70	
bean, adzuki	L	1	
bean, anasazi (Anasazi Native American tribe of southwest)	L	2	
bean, black	L	3	
bean, cannellini	L	4	
bean, fava	L	5	
bean, garbanzo	L	6	

GENERAL PRODUCE--ALL

bean, kidney	L	7
bean, mung	L	8
lentils, brown	L	9
lentils, French green	L	10
lentils, red	L	11
peanuts (underground legume)	L	12
soybean, edamame, miso, tofu	L	13
split pea, yellow	L	14
split pea, green	L	15
almond	N	1
Brazil nut	N	2
cashew	N	3
chestnuts	N	4
coconut	N	5
filberts/hazelnuts	N	6
macadamia nut	N	7
pecans	N	8
pine nuts (a.k.a. pinoli or pignon)	N	9
pistachio	N	10
walnuts, black (Juglans nigra)	N	11
walnuts, English	N	12
apricot	OIL	1
avocado oil	OIL	2
coconut	OIL	3
olive oil	OIL	4
peanut	OIL	5
sesame	OIL	6
walnut	OIL	7
allspice	S	1
black pepper (Piper nigrum)	S	2
capers	S	3
caraway seed	S	4
cardamom	S	5
cinnamon (Cinnamomum verum, C. cassia)	S	6
cloves (Syzygium aromaticum)	S	7
coriander (cilantro seed)	S	8
cumin (Cuminum cyminum)	S	9
ginger	S	10
lemon-pepper	S	11
mace (skin of nutmeg shell)	S	12
mustard seed	S	13
nutmeg	S	14
paprika	S	15
star anise (Illicium verum)	S	16
tamarind (Tamarindus indica)	S	17
turmeric (Cucuma longa)	S	18
chia seeds	Sd	1
Flax (Linum usitatissimum) gold, brown	Sd	2
poppy (Papaver rhoeas, Escholzia californica)	Sd	3
pumpkin seeds	Sd	4
sesame seed	Sd	5
sunflower seed (Helianthus)	Sd	6

GENERAL PRODUCE--ALL

arame	SEA	1
dulse	SEA	2
hijiki	SEA	3
kelp	SEA	4
kombu	SEA	5
Nori	SEA	6
wakame	SEA	7
horsetail (Equisetum arvense)	SKIN	
Witch hazel (Hamamelis virginiana)	SKIN	
cacao (Theobroma cacao)	Sw	
carob, flour	Sw	
stevia (rebaudiana)	Sw	
chamomile (Matricaria recutita)	Tea H	
St. John's Wort (Hypericum perforatum)	Mood H	
Ginkgo biloba	Brain H	
arnica (Arnica montana Asteraceae)	TOPICAL	
comfrey (Symphytum officinale)	TOPICAL	
artichoke, globe (Asteraceae compositae)	V	1
artichoke, Jerusalem (rhizome)	V	2
asparagus	V	3
avocados	V	4
bamboo	V	5
beet	V	6
beet greens	V	7
Bok Choy	V	8
broccoli	V	9
broccoli raab, broccolini	V	10
brussels sprouts	V	11
cabbage, green	V	12
cabbage, Napa (Chinese)	V	13
cabbage, red	V	14
cabbage, savoy	V	15
carrots	V	16
cauliflower	V	17
celeriac (Apiaceae graveolens)	V	18
celery (stalk, leaves, seeds)	V	19
chicory	V	20
collards	V	21
corn	V	22
cucumber	V	23
Daikon radish	V	24
eggplant	V	25
fennel (bulbous base, fern-like leaves, celery-like stalk	V	26
green beans [haricot vert] (Fabaceae)	V	27
Hubbard squash (winter squash)	V	28
jicama	V	29
kale (Blue/Scotch, Purple/Red, Lacinato(Italian)	V	30
kohlrabi	V	31
leek	V	32
lettuce, arugula (rocket) (Eruca sativa)	V	33
lettuce, Belgian Endive	V	34
lettuce, Boston/Bibb lettuce	V	35

GENERAL PRODUCE--ALL

lettuce, buttercup	v	36
lettuce, curly leaf Endive	v	37
lettuce, escarole	v	38
lettuce, loose leaf	v	39
lettuce, radicchio	v	40
lettuce, Red Leaf	v	41
lettuce, romaine	v	42
lettuce, sorrel(Rumex acetosa,et al)	v	43
lettuce, treviso ("oval version" of radicchio)	v	44
mesclun (early spring greens mix)	v	45
mustard greens	v	46
okra	v	47
olives (Halkidiki,Cerignola,Kalamata,Castelvetrano,Beldi,Ascolana)	v	48
onion, shallot	v	49
onion, Spanish	v	50
onion, yellow	v	51
onions, red	v	52
onions,green (a.k.a. scallions)	v	53
parsnip	v	54
pea, snowpea	v	55
peas, garden	v	56
peas, sugar snap	v	57
pepper, Anaheim	v	58
pepper, bell (yellow, red, orange, etc.)	v	59
pepper, cayenne	v	60
pepper, Habanero	v	61
pepper, Hungarian wax	v	62
pepper, Jalapeno	v	63
pepper, Poblano	v	64
pepper, Red Fresno	v	65
pepper, Shishito	v	66
pepper, Szechuan	v	67
pepper, Thai chili	v	68
plantain	v	69
potato, Russet	v	70
potatoes, blue	v	71
potatoes, Yukon Gold	v	72
potatoes, red	v	73
pumpkin	v	74
radish, icicle	v	75
radish, red	v	76
rhubarb	v	77
spinach	v	78
sprouts (seeds, legumes, etc.)	v	79
squash, acorn (winter)	v	80
squash, butternut (winter)	v	81
squash, Chayote (Seculum edule) (summer squash)	v	82
squash, spaghetti	v	83
squash, zucchini	v	84
squash,yellow (crookneck)	v	85
sunchoke	v	86
sweet potato	v	87

Olives:
(Greek: Halkidiki, Kalamata
Italian: Cerignola, Castelvetrano
Peruvian: Ascolana

GENERAL PRODUCE--ALL

Swiss Chard	V	88
taro root	V	89
tomatillo (related to tomato)	V	90
tomatoes, red	V	91
tomatoes, yellow & other	V	92
turnip root	V	93
turnip greens	V	94
water chestnuts	V	95
Watercress (Nasturtium officinale)	V	96
yam (use without skin)	V	97
mushroom-button	V-MYCO	1
mushroom-crimini	V-MYCO	2
mushroom-enoki	V-MYCO	3
mushroom-morel	V-MYCO	4
mushroom-oyster	V-MYCO	5
mushroom-porcini	V-MYCO	6
mushroom-Portabello	V-MYCO	7
mushroom-shiitake	V-MYCO	8
total count	**327**	

Flavors of the World (Eof HS&F)

Africa	peppercorns, cardamom, allspice,cinnamon,cloves,ginger,turmeric,lavender,rosebuds, fennel, etc.
Caribbean	Creole (tomatoes, onions, peppers), ginger, allspice, mango, Jamaican jerk sauce, etc.
West/Northern Europe	chocolate, rosehips, cabbage, endive, Black Forest cake, Danishes, potato, etc.
Eastern Europe/Russia	poppy seed, onions, tomatoes, cabbage, root vegetables, spinach, paprika, buckwheat..

>**Borscht (soup)**: beets, garlic, spinach, carrots, etc.
>**Kolachi**: raised-dough pastry with fruit and/or poppy seeds, walnuts, honey
>**Kapusta Halushki**: cabbage in potato dumpling
Palatsinki: crepes with plum butter and poppy seeds
Pierogis: noodle dough ravioli-like pastry with plums

Greece & Turkey — feta, grape leaves, grapes, oregano, pistachios,pita bread, rice, rosewater, saffron, spinach, sunflower seeds, tomatoes, watermelon, white beans, pine nuts, rice, dill, etc.
>**Moussaka**: eggplant, ground lamb or beef, seasoned sauce
>**Tzatziki**: yogurt w/cucumber, mint, garlic, typically used for gyro("heedo") sandwiches
>**Borek**: pastries stuffed w/spinach
>**Imam Bayildi**: eggplant stuffed w/onion, tomatoes, garlic
>**Rahat Loukoum/Turkish Delight**: heavy sugar syrup, rosewater, cornstarch, mastic

Mediterranean Europe — France, Spain, Italy
figs, olives, artichokes, melon, fennel, herbs, garlic, onions, tomatoes, nuts, squash, …
Paella (Sp.): vegetables, seafood, meat and rice, seasoned with saffron
Ratatouille (Fr.): eggplant, tomatoes, green peppers & squash, etc.
Tapenade: spread of usually olives, capers & anchovies; also artichokes

Middle East — Allspice, basil, bulgur, caraway, cardamom,cassia,chick peas, chilies, cilantro, coriander, cinnamon, cloves, cumin, dill, eggplant, fennel, fenugreek, figs, garlic, ginger, honey, lemon, marjoram, mint, olives, orange-flower water, parsley, phyllo pastry, pine nuts, pomegranates, rosemary, saffron, sesame, tahini, thyme, turmeric, yogurt
>**Tabbouleh**: chopped parsley, tomatoes, onions, bulgur, lemon juice, olive oil
>**Hummus bi Tahina**: pureed chick peas blended w/tahini
>**Moutabal**: smoked pureed eggplants
>**Ful Medames**:(Egypt) fava beans in cold dressing of lemon,garlic,cumin,onion,olive oil
>**Labaneya**:(Egypt) Spinach soup w/yogurt
>**Kadaif**: Shredded pastry dough cake stuffed w/honey syrup & chopped nuts(baklava?)
>**Ma'amoul**:(Syria & Lebanon) nut or date-filled pastries
Baba Ghannouj: eggplant, lemon,tahini, parsley,olive oil

India, Bangladesh	Andhra Pradesh, Bengali, Madras, etc.--curry, masala, tandoori, cardamom, etc.,
Mexico,C. & S. America	epazote(bitter herb for tenderizing beans),masa harina, beans, corn, tortillas, etc.
North America	crabapples (reportedly only plant "native" to North America), etc. (melting pot of world) turkey, cranberry, peach, etc.
South America	Guatemala--avocado, cacao, coffee bean, chia seed, quinoa, papaya, etc.
China	Szechuan, Mandarin, Cantonese, Pekingese--Szechuan pepper, dim sum, etc.
Japan	wasabi radish, shiitake, enoki, and other mushrooms
Korea	kim chi
Polynesia, Indonesia	Tahiti(Noni fruit), kava, etc.
Taiwan	black fungus mushroom
Thailand	Thai chile pepper, Thai red rice, lemongrass
Vietnam	Vietnamese cinnamon
Ceylon	Ceylon cinnamon

Appetizers, Snacks & Sandwiches

Preparation Tips

Avocados: using a paring knife, with the avocado either resting on a cutting board (or for those more experienced), or resting in your hand, cut the avocado from top to bottom, returning to the top. With the paring knife, or a chef knife, press the knife blade flat into the avocado pit/seed until you can turn the seed, then twist until it comes out. Discard the seed, and either slice the avocado, or use a spoon to scoop out the flesh. If slicing the avocado, peel off the skin after slicing.

Kiwifruit: for smoothies, cut fruit across with a spoon, and scoop out both halves. For slices, use paring or other sharp knife to slice to desired thickness, then peel off skin.

Kumquats: can be eaten whole

Feijoa, Passion Fruit & Guava: slice in half, and scoop out insides. Guava has large non-edible garlic-shaped pit in middle, peel around this.

Papaya: slice lengthwise, clean out black seeds, and scoop out flesh with spoon. May also peel skin, but this may take longer, and requires sharp-bladed peeler.

Asian Pear: remove core as with pears and apples.

Pomegranate: peel off skin, remove white pith around arils, scoop out arils--only arils can be eaten.

Rambutan: cut in half, squeeze out & eat white flesh(somewhat astringent/drying), leave out yellowish seed in middle

Starfruit: rinse, slice and eat! Skin and flesh are edible and delicious!

Carambola: cut in half, scoop out and eat aromatic white flesh, and discard hard black seeds.

Appetizers, Snacks & Sandwiches

1 5-layer Guacamole Bean Dip

5	avocados (skin slightly gives to pressure), mashed (remove seed and skin)
2	large tomatoes, diced 1/4 inch, remove stem core
1 Tbsp	juice of 1 lime (Tip: roll and knead lime to extract as much juice as possible)
2 Tbsp	cilantro, chopped (1/4 cup if fresh)
4 oz	white onion, diced 1/4 inch
3 cloves	garlic, minced
1/4 tsp	coriander powder
1/4 tsp	cumin
45 oz	refried, or pinto beans, mashed
30 oz	black, and/or Spanish olives
1/2 cup	tomatoes, diced 1/4 inch, for garnish
1/4 cup	green onions, sliced 1/4 inch
1 lb.	yellow, blue and red tortilla chips
	sea salt to taste (if desired)

In a 4-qt bowl, combine avocados, tomatoes, lime juice, cilantro, garlic & onion until thoroughly mixed. Add coriander and cumin to beans, and mix well. Place mashed pinto beans into casserole or desired serving dish, spread until even. Add guacamole mixture on top of beans, and spread until even. Garnish with olives, tomatoes and green onions, and additional cilantro if desired. Serve with tortilla chips, vegetables, etc.
Makes about 15 cups.

2 Fluted Stuffed Mushrooms

10	button (common) mushrooms
1	garlic clove, minced
2 Tbsp	pine nuts
1	celery rib w/ leaves
	extra-virgin olive oil, chilled
1/2	red bell pepper, finely shredded
1 Tbsp	capers

Using paring knife, flute mushrooms (slightly peel) to achieve a pinwheel design from bottom rim of cap to top of cap. Combine garlic, pine nuts, olive oil, celery with leaves, and red pepper, and hand-mix with spoon until well-blended. Spoon mixture evenly into mushrooms. Serve warm.
Serves 10

3 Funghi con pinoli (mushrooms with pine nuts) (adapted from <u>Classic Italian Cooking</u>)

4	Portabello mushrooms, stem removed
1 c	pine nuts
4	garlic cloves, minced
1/4 c	extra virgin olive oil
1	medium zucchini (8-10 inches long)(20-25cm), grated
1	red onion, diced 1/4 inch, or bunch of green onions(scallions) sliced 1/4 inch
1 bunch	green onions sliced 1/4 inch
6" sprig	rosemary, garnish

Combine pine nuts, garlic, olive oil, zucchini, and onions, mix thoroughly. Spoon mixture evenly into Portabellos. Garnish with rosemary and remainder of green onions. Serve warm. Serves 4-8.

Appetizers, Snacks & Sandwiches

4 Potato Wedges   8.4.2013

4 medium	red potatoes
1 cup	light olive oil for frying
1/2 cup	natural creamy honey mustard dressing, w/o HFCS or artificial colors (see *Dressings*)
2 Tbsp	ground flaxseed
1/2 tsp	yellow mustard powder
1/2 tsp	turmeric
2 tsp	Mrs. Dash Table Blend
1 tsp	paprika
1 tsp	onion powder
1/8 cup	honey

Preheat oven to 350 degrees on "Bake".
Wash and de-eye potatoes, slice in half lengthwise, then slice halves into 3 pieces each. Combine remainder of ingredients, mix until smooth, and place potato slices into mixture, to completely coat, then place onto 12"x18" cookie sheet or pan with at least 1 inch rims. Bake in 350 degree oven for 15 minutes, turn pan around, and broil for 5-10 minutes or until dark golden brown.

5 Spinach-Artichoke Dip--a national favorite revised to another favorite

30 oz frozen	spinach
10 oz (20)	artichoke hearts (jar, or fresh)
1 cup	pine nuts, minced
16 oz	extra virgin olive oil
8 cloves	garlic, minced
8 oz	vegan creamy/cheesy substance (Lisanatti almond mozzarella, for example)

Thaw frozen spinach, or thinly slice 5 oz raw spinach leaves. Combine spinach, pine nuts, artichoke hearts, and garlic in a 5-quart mixer bowl. Using paddle on 1st speed, beat until blended, or stir well with spoon. Add olive oil, and blend on speed 2 or 3 until creamy. Add vegan creamy/cheesy substance if desired (to add creaminess/"cheesiness"). Mix in, and serve. No heating necessary.   Makes at least 1.5 quarts, or 1 9x13 pan.

6 Stuffed Cabbage

1 c	long grain brown rice
1 c	buckwheat groats
2	garlic cloves, minced (about 1 Tbsp)
2	Roma (plum) tomatoes, crushed
1/2 tsp	paprika
1/2 tsp	coriander
4 large(6-8")	green cabbage leaves
1/4 c	white onion or green onions, chopped
1/2 tsp	oregano
	heated marinara sauce for "cover sauce"

Combine rice and buckwheat in 2-quart saucepan, rinse with cool water once, fill to 1 inch above mixture, bring to boil, reduce heat and cook on medium-high for 15 minutes. Add half of paprika, coriander, onions, tomatoes and oregano to mixture, cook another 10 minutes until grains are cooked but not mushy, and vegetables are tender.
While grains are cooking, bring 6- or 8- quart pan of cool water to half-boil on medium heat. Blanch cabbage leaves until soft and workable without breaking, about 20-30 minutes.
Place 1/3 - 1/2 cup of cooked grain-vegetable mixture onto center of cabbage leaf, fold in the sides, and roll up to seal the mixture in, and set aside so joint is on the bottom.

Appetizers, Snacks & Sandwiches

7   Stuffed Peppers
- 2   red, yellow or orange bell peppers
- 4   porcini mushrooms
- 2 Tbsp   fennel seed
- 6 Tbsp   pine nuts, walnuts, almonds, or pistachios, etc.
- 1/2 c   red onion, diced
- 1 tsp   dill weed
- 1/2 c   sun-dried tomatoes (in olive oil)
- 1/2 tsp   sage, rubbed
- 1/2 cup   artichoke hearts or asparagus

Cut top 3/4 inch off peppers, and remove seeds and white "pith". Dice onions, mushrooms, tomatoes and artichokes/asparagus. Mix mushrooms, onion, tomatoes, dill, fennel, sage artichokes/asparagus and nuts until well-blended, using a whisk or food processor.
Split evenly into 2 portions, 1 for each pepper. Using a spoon, spatula, or pastry bag, put half of mixture into each pepper, filling to the rim and above as necessary according to how much mixture you have. Makes 3 cups of stuffing mixture, divided by 2 peppers, is 1 1/2 cups mixture per pepper.

8   Ukrainian Xlopse(my version), a.k.a. Stuffed Cabbage
- 8   green cabbage leaves
- 2 cups   long grain brown rice
- 1 cup   buckwheat groats
- 2 cups   tomato puree
- 2 Tbsp   fennel seed
- 2 Tbsp   parsley, fresh, chopped
- 1 Tbsp   coriander seed powder
- 2 Tbsp   paprika (Hungarian paprika, if possible)
- 1 tsp   black pepper

Combine rice and buckwheat in 2-quart saucepan, rinse with cool water once, fill to 1 inch above mixture, bring to boil, reduce heat and cook on medium-high for 15 minutes. Add half of paprika, coriander, fennel, parsley, and pepper to mixture, cook another 10 minutes until grains are cooked but not mushy, and vegetables are tender.
In a separate 1-quart saucepan, warm tomato puree on medium-low heat, and stir in 1/2 the herbs and spices.
While grains are cooking, bring 6- or 8- quart pan of cool water to half-boil on medium heat. Blanch cabbage leaves until soft and workable without breaking, about 20-30 minutes.
Place 1/3 - 1/2 cup of cooked grain-vegetable mixture onto center of cabbage leaf, fold in the sides, and roll up to seal the mixture in, and set aside so joint is on the bottom.

Rice Pilaf:

There are two (2) types of rice pilaf: the cooking method, and the ingredient content, and/or the mixture name. Typically, most classical recipe books will teach you that "rice pilaf" is made by sautéing the rice with some sort of stock [meat base, or mirepoix (carrots, celery & onions) mixed into a gallon or so of water]. There are also rice pilafs that have rice and orzo (wheat pasta shaped like a sharp-pointed oval), which, in my opinion, is very deceptive, since they are hiding wheat in an otherwise rice-based mixture.

Merriam-Webster's Collegiate Dictionary, 11th edition, defines pilaf as:

> (from Turkish and Persian origin [pilav].) A dish made of seasoned rice and often meat.

The "*old world pilaf*" used in this book was named by someone possibly at Lundberg Farms, which is famous for its Eco-farmed and organic rice production. Thus, the author uses this brand primarily. ***This particular blend includes*** : **long grain brown rice, red wehani rice (also called "Thai red rice"), black japonica rice, wild rice bits, red, green and brown lentils, yellow & green split peas, & black-eye peas.** Quite the satisfying meal, and you can season it any way you like, since it is sold in bulk, and thus there is no seasoning packet with so many strange ingredients such as those found in store-bought or foodservice rice boxes.

Typically, the method I use for cooking rice, including this blend, is either cooking it for 30-45 minutes on medium-high or so, OR, soaking the mixture for an hour or so (while you're busy doing other things), then when you're ready, turn the heat on for about 15 minutes to warm it up, remove it from the heat, mix in any vegetables, seasonings, etc., you want in there, and serve. Basically, put some in a sauce pan, rinse a couple times under cool running water to get the residue out, and put it on the burner. 30 minutes is the typical time to cook, however, sometimes altitude or other factors suggest some extra time. If you're cooking beans with this blend, 30 minutes of cooking works pretty good, especially garbanzo and black. Pinto beans require extra time soaking, though! For the traditional method: saute garlic and/or onions in oil until golden-brown, add rice, saute mixture until rice is soft and almost chewy, and somewhere in this process add your seasonings, stock/mirepoix, etc. This is different with every cook, depending on the intended finished product. **Tip for garlic lovers:** the beneficial chemistry of garlic gets destroyed by heat, so, go ahead and sauté your garlic, but then at the end, slice or mince some cloves, mix them in after cooking, before serving; that way you have both the flavor AND the benefits!   **Adding frozen vegetables in the last 5-10 minutes of the cooking process produces the best results.*

Purple Rice   Another interesting rice used in this book is "Emperor's Rice", (sold by Lotus Foods, etc.), is a dark purplish rice, typically eaten only by the "Emperor" of whatever Asian province, & "forbidden" to everyone else, supposedly because the purple rice is richer in nutrients.

Ginger root: may be eaten whole with skin, or peeled. (peeling may be aggravating (or injurious) with such a small object)

Garlic: For further reference in this book, garlic is typically referred to as "cloves", or the individual "pieces" of the head of garlic. Not to be confused with the SPICE called "clove".

- Large: about thumb size (somewhat rare). Or use 2 medium-size cloves
- Medium: size between index finger and little finger
- Small: less than 1/2" (about 1 cm) wide

Beans Rice & Grains Tips

Cooking Information for Beans and Grains

Name (1 cup dry)	Water needed (cups)	Cooking Time (minutes)	Approx. Yield (cups)
Amaranth	2.5-3	20-25	2 1/2
Buckwheat groats	2	15-25	2 1/2
Millet	2.5-3	35-40	3 1/2
Oat groats**	2	45-60	3
Steel-cut oats**	4	40-45	3
Rolled Oats	1 1/2	10	2 1/2
Rice, brown	2-2.5	30-45	2-2.5
Rice, wild	2.5 - 3	45-50	2.5-3
Quinoa	2	15	3

** Soak overnight to reduce cooking time

Name	Water needed (cups)	Cooking Time (minutes)	Approx. Yield (cups)
Adzuki (Aduki)	4	45-55	3
Anasazi	2.5-3	45-55	2.25
Black Beans	4	60-90	2.25
Black-eyed Peas	3	60	2
Cannellini (White Kidney)	3	45	2.5
Cranberry Bean	3	40-45	3
Fava Beans, skins removed	3	40-50	1 2/3
Garbanzos (chick peas)	4	1 - 3 hrs	2
Great Northern beans	3.5	90	2 2/3
Green Split Peas	4	45	2
Yellow Split Peas	4	60-90	2
Green Peas, whole	6	60-120	2
Kidney Beans	3	60	2.25
Lentils, brown	2.25	45-60	2.25
Lentils, green	2	30-45	2
Lentils, red	3	20-30	2-2.5
Lima Beans, large	4	45-60	2
Lima Beans, small	4	50-60	3
Lima Beans, Christmas	4	60	2
Mung Beans	2.5	60	2
Navy Beans	3	45-60	2 2/3
Pink Beans	3	50-60	2.75
Pinto Beans	3	60-90	2 2/3
Soybeans	4	3 - 4 hrs	3

Beans, Rice & Grains

1 Adzuki and Jasmine Rice Pilaf
- 2 c — brown jasmine rice, uncooked (Lundberg)
- 2 c — adzuki beans, dry
- 1 oz — ginger root
- 1/2 oz — shiitake mushrooms (dried)
- 16 oz — sesame oil (untoasted)
- 1/2 c — cilantro, fresh
- 1/4 c — 5-spice powder
- 1/4 c — Ginkgo biloba leaf, dried
- 1/8 tsp — cayenne pepper, or Szechuan pepper
- 2 — garlic cloves, minced
- 1/2 tsp — red chili pepper, dried, finely chopped
- 1/2 c — mung bean sprouts

Rinse & cook jasmine rice and adzuki beans in 7 cups cool water for 30 minutes on medium heat. Soak shiitake mushrooms in warm water for 15 minutes. Combine ginger root, cilantro, 5-spice, Ginkgo biloba, cayenne/Szechuan pepper, chili pepper, garlic & 6 oz sesame oil in a 1-quart bowl until well-blended. When rice is done, add mushrooms and spice-oil blend, add mung bean sprouts, and stir together until well-blended, or as an option, add the mushrooms as a garnish. Add oil to preferred taste or moisture level. Makes at least 6 cups.

2 Asian Rice 7.24.2017
- long-grain brown rice
- coconut oil
- olive oil
- Thai Kitchen red curry paste
- Thai Kitchen green curry paste
- fresh ginger root
- carrots
- Kim Chi (Jo San), mild or hot, depending on your taste buds
- red onion
- horseradish mustard
- 2 garlic cloves
- sesame seeds
- broccoli florets (steamed)
- sunflower seeds
- 50-50 blend greens (spinach, kale, chard)
- fresh mushrooms (button, shiitake, etc.)
- bean sprouts (mung or black)
- sliced almonds
- splash of organic lemon juice (approx. 1 Tbsp)
- turmeric

Beans, Rice & Grains

3 Best Rice & Vegetable Pilaf

1 cup	long grain brown rice
1/2 cup	Old World Pilaf Lundberg rice-legume blend
1/2 cup	black beans
2 cups	red cabbage, 1/2" julienne strips
1	Roma tomato, diced
1 cup	snow peas, halved & trimmed
2	carrots, grated
1 cup	coleslaw mix (dry)
3/4 cup +	olive oil
1/8 tsp	coriander
1/8 tsp	cumin
1/8 tsp	ginger powder
1 Tbsp	oregano
1 tsp	cilantro leaves, dry
1/8 cup	fresh cilantro leaves, chopped or torn coarsely
1/8 cup	green onions, 1/4" chopped
1/4 cup +	Bragg Liquid Aminos

To cook: (grain method) place rice, rice pilaf blend and black beans into 2-quart saucepan, rinse, add 2 1/2 cups water, set heat on medium-high, & cook for 30 minutes. Stir in spices and herbs. In a 2-quart bowl, combine cabbage, tomato, carrots, coleslaw mix, olive oil, green onions, and 1/8 cup Liquid Aminos, and stir together until well-blended. Combine rice mixture and vegetable mixture, add oil and Liquid Aminos to taste, garnish with snow peas, cilantro and tomato. Makes about 9 cups.

4 Goddess Lentils and Spinach Rice Pilaf   [makes about 1 gallon]

1/2 cup	short grain brown rice
1/4 cup	buckwheat groats
1/4 cup	French green lentils
2	beets, 1/4" dice
1	black radish, grated
5 oz	spinach
1/3 cup	red onion, 1/8" slice
1/3 cup	Simple Truth organic Goddess Dressing
3 Tbsp	golden flax seed
3	crimini mushrooms, 1/8" sliced
	carrots, 1/8" coins
15 oz can	black beans
1	shishito pepper, minced
1 Tbsp	ginger root, grated
1/2 tsp	cardamom powder
2 Tbsp	oregano
2 Tbsp	cumin
1 tsp	coriander
4 Tbsp	sage
1 tsp	5-spice powder
	(avocado)
	"Thai Peanut Satay" sauce
	olive oil

Directions: Cook rice, lentils and buckwheat with olive oil for 30 minutes. Add herbs & flax when rice is done cooking. Prepare vegetables and place into large bowl. Combine vegetables with rice mixture, add sauces, stirring until well-blended.

5 Honey-Mustard Rice Pilaf

1/4 cup	old world pilaf
1/8 cup	millet
1/8 cup	wild rice blend
1 Tbsp	wild rice
1/4 cup	garbanzo beans
1/4 cup	black-eye peas
2 cups	broccoli, 1 inch or smaller pieces
2	carrots, sliced 1/8"
1/8 cup	white onion, minced
1 cup	pecans (1/2 in mixture, 1/2 topping)
1 Tbsp	Italian seasoning
1 tsp	sage, rubbed
1 Tbsp	parsley flakes
1/8 cup	honey mustard
1 tsp	garlic powder
1 Tbsp	Bragg's Liquid Aminos
6 large	romaine lettuce leaves, 1/2 inch strips
1 8-oz can	mandarin oranges (or 2 whole fresh mandarin oranges), for garnish
1 16-oz can	crushed pineapple, for garnish

Cook grains and beans for 20-30 minutes. Slice carrots and chop broccoli into 1 inch pieces, then steam broccoli and carrots for 5-7 minutes in separate 6" pan with 1/2 inch of water, and add onions 3 minutes later. Add herbs to rice in last 10 minutes of cooking. Combine onion, 1/2 of pecans, romaine, Liquid Aminos and honey mustard, and blend together. Combine the vegetables and rice mixture, garnish with mandarins, remaining half of pecans and pineapple. Makes about 10 cups (about 2 1/2 quarts).

6 Jambalaya Rice & Beans 7.17.2017 (dairy-free & gluten-free)

1 cup	long grain brown rice	
3	garlic cloves	
2	Andouille sausage links, par-cooked & sliced	
3	carrots (1at beginning, 2 near end of cooking)	**Mirepoix**
1/2 cup	red onion	
1	1 green onion	
1 stalk	celery	
5	collard leaves, julienne & halved	
1 stalk	fresh dill, chopped	
1	red bell pepper	
1/8 cup	fresh ginger, sliced & chopped	
15 oz can	black beans	
1/8 cup	flaxseed meal, added after cooking, to soak up excess liquid	
1/8 tsp	cayenne	
1 Tbsp	lemon shot (org. lemon juice & lemon oil)	
1/2 cup	coconut oil	

Beans, Rice & Grains

7 Italian Vegetable Risotto

14 oz	dry Lundberg Wild Rice blend, or brown (whole grain) Arborio Rice
6 oz	artichoke hearts
2 1/2	carrots, sliced
1/2 cup	red or white onion, sliced 1/4" x 1" julienne
1/2 head	curly Endive lettuce or Romaine, 3/4" x 1-1/2" strips
16 oz	garbanzo or cannellini beans
3	garlic cloves, thinly sliced
1/8 cup	Italian seasoning
1 Tbsp	pizza seasoning
6 oz	pesto (dairy-free)
12 oz	Italian Herb marinara sauce
	olive oil (light for sautéing) or non-dairy butter
2 pints (32 oz)	vegetable stock

Directions: Sweat onions in 1 1/2 oz refined olive oil or butter. Add rice and mix thoroughly with butter or oil. Cook it, stirring occasionally, until a toasted aroma develops. Add 1/3 of vegetable stock, stirring rice every few minutes until rice absorbs the Add remaining stock in 2 more additions, stirring frequently. Cook risotto until rice is al dente and liquid is mostly absorbed, and texture is creamy. Cook beans in a separate pan while cooking risotto. When risotto and beans are done, stir in vegetables, garlic, herbs and pesto. Ladle marinara sauce over mixture prior to serving.

8 Lemon-Ginger Lentils   7.15.2013 dinner

8 large	romaine leaves
16 oz	chick peas
16 oz	brown lentils or split peas
2 Tbsp	lemon-ginger tea mix (bulk-lemongrass, ginger, coriander seed,...)
8 oz	brown jasmine rice
2 Tbsp	minced garlic
3 full cups	baby spinach
1 julienned	green bell pepper (or other color)
1/2 cup diced	white onion
1 cup	sugar snap peas
1	sweet potato, sliced in half, thirds, then 1/8" slabs
8 oz	mandarin oranges (garnish)
1/2 cup	slivered almonds (garnish)

(these 3 steamed 5 minutes with celery seed)

Ginger-Peanut Sauce

1/2 cup	peanut butter
1/4 cup	apricot jam or preserves
1/4 cup	Liquid Aminos
1/4 cup	honey
1 tsp	ginger powder, or 2 Tbsp finely-grated ginger root
1 tsp	turmeric
1 tsp	mustard
as needed	olive oil

Directions: Combine chickpeas, lentils, lemon-ginger tea mix, and brown jasmine rice, and cook for 30 minutes on medium heat until soft. Stir in 2 Tbsp oil.
Steam pepper, onion and sugar snap peas with celery seed in sauce pan with 1 cup of water, and snug-fitting lid for 3 minutes, then stir in garlic and spinach. Slice sweet potato, and boil over medium-high heat until fork easily penetrates.

Beans, Rice & Grains

Lemon-ginger Lentils cont'd.
Combine all SAUCE ingredients, and whisk together until smooth and creamy. Shred lettuce into 1/2" x 2" strips, layer on bottom of casserole dish, or platter. Layer chickpea mixture over lettuce, then top with sautéed vegetable-spinach mixture, sweet potato slabs, mandarin oranges, then evenly drizzle with sauce.

9 Mincemeat Breakfast Cereal
1 c	currants or raisins
2	Golden Delicious apples
1 c	buckwheat groats
1 tsp	cloves
1 tsp	cinnamon

Core apples, and chop into 1/4" pieces or smaller. Mix apples, spices and currants into buckwheat groats.

10 Mount Curry   (did for gluten-free/vegetarians @ Sheraton banquet, 5.5.2014) Plated Version

1/2 cup	wild rice blend
1 1/2 cups	brown lentils
2	yellow squash, 1/8" thick by 1/2" wide by ~ 1 1/2" long
1 8"	zucchini, quartered, bias-cut
30 (baby)	carrots(baby used, or regular), cut same as yellow squash
1/2 of 3" onion	red onions, 1/4"-3/8" dice
2 per person	mushrooms(crimini, white, etc.[small]), 1/8" sliced, then coarsely chopped
1 cup/person	spinach (baby spinach preferred), 1/4" sliced
1	red bell pepper, thinly cut (garnish)
	Sauce
4 Tbsp	fennel seed
2 Tbsp	curry powder
2 Tbsp	cumin
2 Tbsp	coriander
3 Tbsp	thyme
3 Tbsp	sage
4 Tbsp	turmeric
1 Tbsp	brown mustard seed
1/2 tsp	cinnamon
3	garlic cloves
1/3 cup packed	cilantro, stemmed and coarsely chopped
dash	cayenne pepper
1 tsp each	sesame seed (garnish)
1 Tbsp each	slivered almonds(garnish)
1 each	cilantro sprigs (garnish)
for rice & sauté	soy-olive oil (or plain olive oil, or sesame oil)

Directions:
1. Cook rice and lentils in twice the water for 30 minutes, with oil and fennel seed. Bring to boil, stir, reduce heat to medium-low, and cover for 20 minutes. Fluff with fork. Add 1/2 of sauce ingredients to rice mixture 10 minutes into cooking.
2. Sauté garlic in oil until golden brown, add mustard seeds, fennel seed.
3. Combine remainder of sauce ingredients in a bowl. Set aside.
4. Add other 1/2 of sauce ingredients to sauté mixture, stirring occasionally, and reduce heat to Low, let simmer while preparing vegetables.
5. Place layer of cut spinach onto plate, leaving a 1 1/2" gap between outside

Beans, Rice & Grains

Mount Curry, cont'd.

and edge of plate. Using a 2-cup clear measuring cup, spoon rice mixture into cup until you have 2 cups, packed. Turn upside down onto center of spinach, and lightly squash mound until about 1 1/2" tall, and round it with your hands, until about 4"- 5" in diameter, and level on top.

6. Sauté the zucchini, mushrooms and red onion in oil, on High heat for about 3 minutes, and using perforated or slotted spoon, scoop vegetables out and lay them around the mound, about an inch high.
7. Carrots and yellow squash: you can either sauté them, or keep them raw. Raw is a little easier to handle. Place carrot & squash slices vertically, leaning up against the mound, all around, kind of like a picture of the sun with its rays.
8. Place the red pepper slices in a radiating pattern from the center of the mound, about 3-6, depending on the slice length. Garnish with sesame, almonds, and place a sprig of cilantro on top in the center.
9. Repeat 5-8 for each plate.

Makes 5 plates.

11 Thai Peanut Satay with Lentils & Vegetables ("Healthy meal for $40) 4.21.2014

French green lentils
artichoke hearts
baked beans
Thai Kitchen peanut Satay sauce
black radish
baby (or regular) carrots
crimini mushrooms
red bell pepper
leek
flaxseed meal
sage, rubbed
ginger
Italian parsley
turmeric

12 Potassium Potpourri (idea from "Potassium" in PNH), dinner 3/2/2013)

1/2 - 1 cup	Old World pilaf
1 1/2 cups	wild rice, uncooked
1/4 cup	black beans, dry
2	avocados, sliced
4	medium (5 inch) sweet potatoes
16	Medjool dates, sliced in 1/2" pieces
1 full sprig	fresh sage, dried
1 1/2 Tbsp	molasses
10	Turkish figs
1/4 cup	pecans, coarsely chopped
4-8 leaves	romaine, cut in 1/2 inch strips, as a "bed"

Cook pilaf, wild rice and black beans for 20-30 minutes until pleasantly chewable. Wash and clean sweet potatoes, put in large pan of boiling water. Cut romaine, and spread out in bottom of 9x13 casserole dish. De-stem figs, and pit and slice dates, and put aside. When rice is done, remove from heat, and remove sweet potatoes from heat, and drain. Cut sweet potatoes in 3/4" cubes, and add to rice mixture. Crumble sage with fingers over rice-potato mixture. Spoon into casserole dish with romaine, and spread out evenly. Top the mixture with figs, dates, pecans and avocado, and drizzle with molasses. Makes a full casserole dish that is delicious and fruity-sweet!

Beans, Rice & Grains

13 Raspberry-Spice Buckwheat Granola

2 lb	buckwheat flakes or groats (soaked)
8 oz	quinoa flakes
4 oz	sesame seeds
1 Tbsp	ginger
1 Tbsp	cinnamon
4 c	raspberries
3/4 c	pumpkin seeds
1 c	cashews
3/4 c	sunflower seeds
1 c	raisins or currants
2 c	almonds
2 c	cranberries, fresh
1 c	pure maple syrup, unsulphured molasses, or agave nectar
1 c	cherries, dried (unsulphured) or fresh

Combine all ingredients and mix together. Serve with nut or rice milk.

14 Red Beans & Rice Crockpot-style   10.29.16   (Pastor Appreciation Sunday)

one-half	yellow onion, chopped
1	green pepper, chopped
1	small shallot, minced
2 lb.	dry long grain brown rice
1	sweet potato, 1/2" cubes
2	15-oz cans red beans
1 tsp	Hungarian paprika
1 Tbsp	ginger root, minced
3 cloves	garlic, minced
1/2 tsp	celery seed
1 cup	brown sugar
1/8 cup	Cadia (or equivalent) coconut oil

Directions: Place all ingredients in 6-quart crockpot with 1-1/2 quarts cold water, and set heat onto HIGH. After 4-6 hours, add 16-32 oz more water or until water level rim of lid.

Reduce heat to LOW, cook another 4 hours and turn off heat. Test doneness of beans. If not serving immediately, refrigerate overnight. Makes 4-6 quarts.

15 Red Lentil Curry Masala   3.23.2014

1 cup	chickpeas, dry
1 cup	red lentils, dry
1/2 cup	red onion, diced
1	red bell pepper, diced in 1/4" x 1"
3	carrots, bias cut
2 Tbsp	fresh garlic cloves, minced
3 tsp	Garam Masala powder
3 tsp	curry powder
1 tsp	cardamom powder
1 tsp	whole fennel seed--grind in mortar & pestle
2/3 cup	raw, shelled pistachios
8 oz	cashews, raw
6 oz	Spicy Nothings Classic Curry medium simmer sauce
3/4 cup	olive oil

1 Rinse and cook chickpeas and lentils together with 1/4 cup of oil on medium for

Page 40

Beans, Rice & Grains

Red Lentil Curry Masala, cont'd.
45 minutes. Prepare vegetables, and combine in 4-qt sauce pan. Combine chickpea mixture with vegetables and remainder of oil, and add spices and curry sauce. Stir well, and add pistachios and cashews, stirring thoroughly.
2 Simmer over low heat for 10-30 minutes, stirring occasionally. Turn off heat and let sit. Serve with rice if desired.   Prep time: about 1-1.5 hours. Makes 10 cups.

16 Red Quinoa & Lentils with Stir-fry Vegetables 5.16.17
green lentils
red quinoa
fresh sage leaves, split & de-stemmed
SOAK ABOVE 3 INGREDIENTS TOGETHER
dried rosemary
ziti or equivalent rice and/or quinoa pasta (Live G-free, etc.)
Cedar's sesame hummus
paprika
Mrs. Dash
Italian seasoning
red radish, sliced
carrot
red beet, sliced + beet greens (stems removed)
Stir-fried in wok:
veg: napa cabbage, olive oil, broccoli & Bok choi, sriracha-sesame ginger sauce, snow peas, turmeric
Sesame-Ginger Sauce ingredients: (pre-packaged)
[sugar], canola oil, sesame oil, soy sauce, distilled vinegar*, sriracha sauce, corn starch, rice vinegar, ginger, pineapple juice, tomato, [sugar], distilled vinegar*, onion, spice, carrots, dried garlic, xanthan gum, spice, paprika, salt, natural flavor, dried peppers, cilantro, xanthan gum, sesame seeds, garlic, spice, [carrageenan, natural flavor], citric acid (use lemon juice)
* substitute apple cider vinegar or rice vinegar

17 Rice & Bean Vegetable Pilaf
4 oz each	black-eyed peas, black beans, pinto beans, kidney beans, lentils, red beans
1 c	wild rice blend (Lundberg)
2	carrots, 8-10" long, sliced
1 c	broccoli flowerets
1 c	mushrooms, sliced (not canned)
1	celery stalk, sliced 1/4"
1	red bell pepper, diced 1/4"
4 oz	artichoke hearts
1 c	spinach leaves
2 tsp	basil
2 tsp	oregano
1 Tbsp	fennel seed
	olive oil

Cook rice and beans with olive oil. Prepare vegetables and combine with rice-bean mixture when cooked. Serve warm.

Beans, Rice & Grains

18 Rice Pilaf, Sheraton (Daughters of American Revolution), seasoning only!
    brown sugar
    tarragon
    turmeric
    sage
    onion powder
    garlic powder
    coriander
    4 oz butter per box of rice
    OR 1/8 c olive oil per box of rice
    (1/2 cup of above seasoning per 2-box pan)

Stir-fry accompanied by above rice (my recipe)
    LaChoy (or equiv.) teriyaki
    sweet soy sauce
    honey
    cream of coconut
    curry
    ginger
    minced garlic (wet), sauteed
    cayenne (1/8 tsp)

19 Rosemary-Red Onion Polenta

6 c	water
3 c	dry polenta
1/2 c	red onion, 1/4" dice
1 sprig	fresh rosemary
1/4 c	pine nuts
6 slices	red onion, sliced 1/4"
Directions:	Bring water to boil, slowly add polenta while stirring, add onions, garlic & 2/3 of rosemary. Reduce heat to medium. Stir to blend, and prevent from sticking or scorching, as mixture becomes very thick. After about 30-40 minutes, polenta should be thick and tough to stir. Remove from heat, and place into 2" half-pan, or square casserole, and let sit 5-10 minutes. Garnish with onion slices and rosemary, and serve. Makes about 9 1-cup servings

Beans, Rice & Grains

20 Supergrain & Fruit Cereal for a month
(the secret here is to buy bags of the grains, and use 2 Tbsp every day)
2 Tbsp	amaranth
2 Tbsp	quinoa (white, red or black)
2 Tbsp	buckwheat groats
2 Tbsp	millet
1 tsp	fresh ginger
1 tsp	cinnamon
1 Tbsp	seedless rosehips
1 Tbsp	golden flaxseed, ground
1 Tbsp	sesame seed
1/3 c mix	fruit: dates, raisins, currants, apricots, berries, figs, or similar fruits
1/3 c mix	macadamia, almonds, pumpkin seeds, walnuts, pecans, sunflower seeds, Brazil, etc.
1/8 c	pure maple syrup, unsulphured molasses, or agave nectar
Directions:	Place amaranth, quinoa, buckwheat, millet, rosehips and cinnamon into 6- or 8 qt. crockpot or slow-cooker, with 1.5 c water, on HIGH for 6-10 hours, or overnight. Turn off heat. Add remaining ingredients of your choice, mix together in slow-cooker, and enjoy! Satisfying and delicious! Makes about 3 cups.

21 Taco-Rice Casserole
1 c	long- or medium-grain brown rice
1 c	pinto beans
1	large tomato
1 head	Romaine lettuce
1 lb.	yellow, blue, and/or red corn tortilla chips (natural)
1	medium onion, diced (red or Spanish)
1 Tbsp	cumin
1 tsp	chili powder
1 Tbsp	cilantro
opt. garnish	guacamole/avocado, olives

Rinse and cook rice and pinto beans (if dry).
Dice tomato into 3/8" cubes, shred Romaine into 1/4" x 1.5" strips, dice onion into 3/8" pieces.
When rice and beans are cooked, stir in cumin, chili powder and cilantro, and layer ingredients on a plate or platter as follows: lettuce, rice-bean mixture, onions, tomatoes, and olives/avocado/guacamole. Garnish with extra cilantro if desired. Serve with tortilla chips. Makes about 11 cups.

Beans, Rice & Grains

22 Tahini-Peanut Satay   4.21.2014

5 oz	Organic Girl Fresh Herbs & Greens
1 gallon	kale
15 oz can	garbanzo beans
1 cup dry	French green lentils, cooked with 2 Tbsp rubbed sage
1/4 cup	buckwheat groats, cooked
1/8 cup	gold flaxseed meal (added to lentils)
20	baby carrots, 1/8" coins
1	red bell pepper, 1/4" dice
1	black radish, 1/4" dice
6	crimini mushrooms, 1/8" sliced
1 cup	loose Italian parsley
3/4 c	Bragg Liquid Aminos
1	leek, 1/4" sliced
1	garlic clove

Sauce

1 2.5"	turmeric root, grated & minced (sauce)
1/8 cup	ginger root, grated & minced (sauce)
8 oz jar	Thai Kitchen peanut Satay sauce (sauce)
1 cup	tahini (sauce)

Directions: Cook lentils, buckwheat and sage together for 30 minutes. Stir in flax when done.
Prepare vegetables and combine in large bowl.
Combine sauce ingredients, stir together until well-blended.
Combine sauce and lentil-buckwheat mixture into vegetable mixture.
Makes about 1 1/2 gallons. Prep time: 2 hrs 10 min.

23 Vegetarian/Vegan Thanksgiving Dinner

1/4 c	wild rice blend (Lundberg), uncooked
1/2 c	pecans
1 tsp	basil
1 tsp	thyme
1 tsp	curry powder
1/4 c	raisins or currants
1 c	cranberries, fresh
1	sweet potato, diced or zested
1/4 c	pure maple syrup, grade A
16 oz	beans (pinto, black, black-eyed peas, red, garbanzo)
1	large red potato, skin-on, mashed or pureed
2	garlic cloves, minced
1/8 c	soymilk or other non-dairy milk
1/2 tsp	parsley
1/2 tsp	chives

Directions: Rinse and cook wild rice and beans in 4 cups water for 30-40 minutes on medium heat, or until slightly chewy. Add herbs in last 10 minutes of cooking. Rinse, peel and boil sweet potato (diced) on medium for 30 minutes, until soft. Steam potato 4 minutes. Place in bowl, mash a few times with potato masher. Add milk until creamy but not liquid, add garlic, chives and parsley.
Whip until thick and creamy. Add pecans, raisins/currants, and cranberries to rice-bean mixture. Pour maple syrup over sweet potato, place prepared potato mixtures next to rice, and serve. Serves 1, or 2 small servings of 1/2-potatoes

Beans, Rice & Grains

24 World Traveler Rice Pilaf   (use your imagination!)
- rice pilaf & legumes
- carrot
- asparagus (or artichoke)
- broccoli
- sweet potato
- celery
- quinoa
- fenugreek
- garlic
- green tea
- oregano
- parsley
- turmeric
- Essiac tea
- flax
- ginger
- cayenne
- coriander
- cumin
- fennel
- peppermint
- black pepper
- cilantro
- cinnamon

25 Dinner Wed. 7.10.2013
- garbanzo beans
- pinto beans
- sugar snap peas
- spinach
- green onions
- white onion
- yellow & green bell pepper
- carrots
- romaine
- wild rice blend
- red quinoa
- Roma tomatoes
- Italian seasoning
- cumin
- coriander
- oregano
- liquid aminos
- poultry seasoning (rosemary, sage, thyme)

Beverages

1 Curative Power Tea   1990's
- 1 Tbsp   black pepper
- 1 Tbsp   lemon pepper seasoning (salt-free)
- 2 Tbsp   fennel seed
- 1/8 c   parsley
- 2 Tbsp   peppermint leaves
- 2 Tbsp   red clover flowers & leaves
- 1 Tbsp   turmeric
- 1 Tbsp   fresh garlic, minced (added 5 minutes after taken off heat)
- 2 Tbsp   chamomile flowers
- 2 Tbsp   burdock root
- 2 Tbsp   calendula officinalis (pot marigold petals)
- 2 Tbsp   dandelion root (organic)
- 2 Tbsp   fenugreek seed

Combine all ingredients except garlic, bring to boil for 10 minutes, remove from heat, let sit for 5 minutes, add garlic, stir, then steep for 15 minutes or longer.

2 Fen 'Beer' 2.14.2014
- fenugreek tea, strong-brewed (ex.: 2 Tbsp in 8 oz water, steeped for 30 minutes)
- Perrier or equiv. mineral water
- apple cider vinegar
- fresh lemon juice (or organic bottled)

3 Fruit Drink
- 1 Tbsp   Bragg Apple Cider Vinegar
- 1 Tbsp   fresh or organic lemon juice
- 6 oz   fresh pineapple juice ****
- 7   cranberries
- 1   peach

Place cranberries, peach and pineapple juice in blender, mix well until smooth. Add cider vinegar and lemon juice, blend for 10-20 seconds. Serve.
****If using whole pineapple, multiply vinegar & lemon juice by 5, triple cranberries & peach

4 Macho Man's Booster Iced Tea (healthy herbal "strong drink")   revised 3/19/2014)
- 1/8 cup   burdock root
- 1/4 c   organic rosehips (seedless if possible)
- 1/8 cup   Ginkgo biloba
- 1/8 cup   pure green tea leaves, preferably organic (bulk tea mix)
- 2 tsp   American, or Korean (Panax) Ginseng
- 1   3" beet, raw, pureed
- 3 Tbsp   freshly squeezed lemon juice
- 1 Tbsp   ginger root
- 1 Tbsp   milk thistle seed, powdered
- 1/4 cup   red clover
- 1/8 tsp   cayenne
- 1 large   garlic clove
- 1 Tbsp   sarsaparilla root
- 1 tsp   saw palmetto
- 1 tsp   Gotu kola
- 1/8 cup   raw apple cider vinegar

Beverages

Macho Man's Booster Iced Tea cont'd
Bring 1 1/2 cups purified water to a boil, add Green Tea, burdock, milk thistle & sarsaparilla root, allow to boil for 1 to 2 minutes. Remove from heat. Let simmer 5 minutes to cool. Place rosehips in lukewarm water & simmer between 20-30 minutes, up to 4 hours for more strength. Strain green tea mixture. Place the following in blender/Vitamix: beet, ginger root, cayenne & garlic. Blend for 2 minutes until smooth, add apple cider vinegar, blend for 10 seconds. Combine rosehip tea, green tea mixture, and blended mixture in blender for 20 seconds. Serve. May add other pure fruit juice if desired.

5 **Pina Colada**
- 1-1/2 cup fresh pineapple
- 1/2 c coconut, flaked (non-sulfured)
- 1/4 c macadamia nuts, raw
- 1 Tbsp fresh ginger

Place all ingredients in blender, mix at high speed for 2 minutes or until smooth. Serve.

6 **Red Tea**
- 1/2 cup red clover
- 1/8 cup hibiscus
- 1/8 cup raspberry-flavored green tea
- 1/8 cup rose hips

For pot: place herbs except rosehips into pot, add at least 1 cup water, bring to boil. Remove from heat. Steep for 10-30 minutes(until desired strength). Add rosehips when liquid is lukewarm. (heat destroys vitamin C). Steep another 30 minutes or longer for rosehips to assimilate. Drink cool or lukewarm. Add ice for a refreshing drink if desired. As an alternative, make suntea with this mixture. Use a 1-2 gallon suntea jar, or even a Mason jar works just as well. Add a sunny window and up to 4 hours of good sunshine.

7 **Strong Drink for Toxic People**
- 1 Tbsp garlic cloves
- 1/2 cup raw apple cider vinegar
- 1/2 cup lemon juice
- 1/8 cup honey (opt.) or other natural sweetener

Mix thoroughly in blender for 1 minute. Drink slowly.

Beverages

8 Summer Fruit Jazz
- 2 (1/8 c) strawberries
- 6 (1/4 c) blueberries
- 1 (1/3 c) kiwifruit (cut in half, scoop out flesh from both halves)
- 1/4 (2 c) fresh pineapple (cut off crown plus 1/2 inch of top, and 1 inch of bottom, peel skin w/knife
- 1/4 c (6) raspberries, rinsed
- 1 (1/4 c) guava (cut in half, scoop out edible flesh inside)
- 1 (2 c) starfruit, quartered (starfruit & carambola are the same fruit +/- one "point")
- 1/4 c pomegranate seeds (arils)
- 1/4 c papaya flesh (no seeds or skin)
- 1 Tbsp raw apple cider vinegar
- 1 Tbsp lemon juice
- 1 Tbsp lime juice
- ice (optional)

Rinse berries, peel pineapple, kiwi, guava, papaya. Throw out any moldy fruit.***
Combine all ingredients in blender (including ice if desired), and blend for
2-5 minutes or until smooth. Makes about 4 cups.

*** Typically, fruit should be firm, especially melons. If flesh is darker than normal, or mushy, throw it out. Ripe kiwifruit is usually mushy and darker green than normal, and has a "sharper" taste. Good kiwifruit is similar in firmness to a good avocado, firm with just a little bit of give.

Breads

1 Gluten-Free New Bread (collaboration with Juli Griffith)
   {This recipe uses a bread machine}
1 c	brown rice flour
1/4 c	buckwheat flour
1/2 c	tapioca flour
1 c	4-flour bean mix (see page 50)****
1/2 c	corn starch
3/4 c	flaxseed egg replacer (1/2 c flax, 2 cups water, blended 2 minutes)
1/2 c	mixed nuts (pecans, walnuts, sunflower seeds…)
1/8 c	cranberries, chopped (fresh or dried unsulphured)
	extra water to mix
2 1/2 tsp	xanthan gum
3/4 c	Celestial Seasonings "Sugar Plum Spice" tea, already brewed
1 Tbsp	bread yeast
3 Tbsp	blackstrap molasses
1/2 tsp	sea salt
1/8 c	hemp seeds or sesame seeds
1/2 tsp	anise seed

Use "dark" setting or "whole grain" setting on bread machine.
**Note: if breadmachine is NOT available, use directions in recipe below

2 GF Seed Bread (idea) for 12" standard size loaf (or could make crackers)
1/8 cup	caraway
1 tsp	celery seed
2 Tbsp	chia
2 Tbsp	cumin
2 Tbsp	fennel
2 Tbsp	fenugreek
4 Tbsp	flaxseed
1 cup	hazelnut/filbert (chopped
4 Tbsp	millet, soaked 1 hour
1 Tbsp	mustard (yellow & brown), soaked 1 hour
4 Tbsp	pumpkin seed
4 Tbsp	quinoa
4 Tbsp	sunflower
4 Tbsp	Flours to use: buckwheat, millet, coconut, almond, gar-fava, amaranth, quinoa
	olive oil
	GF baking yeast
	tapioca starch
	xanthan gum

Breads

3 Hearty Hazelnut GF Bread
- 1 package   Bob's Red Mill GF Hearty Wholegrain Bread Mix"
- [egg alt.]   1/2 c golden flaxseed w/1 cup water, blended 1-2 minutes until thick
- 1 tsp   apple cider vinegar
- 1/3 c   hazelnuts or filberts
- 1 1/2 Tbsp   sesame seeds
- 1/2 Tbsp   caraway seeds
- 1/4 c   almond culinary oil (use for oil in mix)
- 1/4 c   black zante currants
- 1.15 oz pkt Justin's Chocolate Hazelnut butter blend
- 2   star anise pods (stars) {blended with hazelnuts and 1 cup water}

Directions:
1. Dissolve enclosed pack of yeast in 1 3/4 cups warm (110 degrees F), and let stand 5 minutes to foam. Have all ingredients at room temperature.
2. Put all dry ingredients (flour mix, sesame seeds, caraway seeds, currants) into 4- or 5-quart mixing bowl, preferably using a countertop mixer.
3. Add flax-water mixture, oil, cider vinegar, yeast-water mixture, chocolate-hazelnut packet, and hazelnut-star anise mixture.
4. With mixer on low speed, blend all ingredients until smooth. Turn mixer to medium and beat 15 seconds or until mixture thickens slightly. Pour into generously greased 9x5 inch bread pan. Smooth top of dough with wet spatula.
5. Bake at 350 degrees or according to directions on package.
   Using oven mitts, remove from oven, and run a butter knife around the edges of the loaf to separate it from the pan, turn the pan upside down over a wire rack and tap the pan until the loaf comes out. Allow to cool.

4 Unleavened Fruit & Nut "Dense Bread"   12/24/2014
- 1/4 cup   buckwheat flour (Arrowhead Mills)
- 2 cups   Bob's Red Mill Sorghum flour
- 1/2 cup   Glutino gluten-free flour (or substitute sorghum flour if you don't like white rice)

Sift above into 4-cup measuring container

- 5/8 cup   pure coconut oil
- 1/2 cup   olive oil
- 3/4 cup   applesauce
- 1/4 cup   flaxseed meal
- 1/8 cup   brown sugar
- 1/2 cup   unsulphured molasses
- 2 tsp   anise seed, crushed with mortar and pestle
- 2 tsp   cinnamon
- 1/3 cup   cranberries
- 1 cup   walnuts (1/3 chopped)
- 1/4 cup   pecans
- 1/4 cup   shredded coconut (unsulphured)
- 3/4 tsp   pure vanilla extract
- 2 Tbsp   pureed plums
- 2 oz   dairy-free 60% cacao mint chocolate, grated
- 1 tsp   orange zest
- 1/8 cup   pure maple syrup

Unleavened Fruit & Nut "Dense Bread" cont'd

Breads

Pour sifted flour into 2-quart mixing bowl, add remainder of ingredients, and mix with wooden spoon until blended and thick.(if using xanthan gum, sift with other dry ingredients). Oil 9x9 casserole dish with olive oil, and spoon mixture into dish, and smooth top so it is level, and corners are filled. Cover in foil, and bake at 350 degrees for 20 minutes. Remove foil, and bake another 20 minutes. Broil for for 5-10 minutes and remove from oven. Serve. Rich, moist and somewhat crumbly. Might add 1/2 teaspoon of xanthan gum to "hold things together" better.

Bette Hagman's Gluten-free Flour Mix Formulas [Gluten-free Gourmet Bakes Bread, p.40]

	For 9 cups	For 12 cups
Gluten-free Flour Mix(original rice mix)		
Rice flour (2 parts)	6 cups	8 cups
Potato starch (2/3 part)	2 cups	2 2/3 cups
Tapioca flour (1/3 part)	1 cup	1 1/3 cup
Light Bean Flour Mix (from Fast & Healthy)		
Garfava bean flour (1 part) [from Authentic Foods]	3 cups	4 cups
Tapioca flour (1 part)	3 cups	4 cups
Cornstarch (1 part)	3 cups	4 cups
**** Four Flour Bean Mix		
Garfava bean flour (2/3 part)	2 cups	2 2/3 cups
Sorghum flour (1/3 part)	1 cup	1 1/3 cups
Cornstarch (1 part)	3 cups	4 cups
Tapioca flour (1 part)	3 cups	4 cups
Featherlight Rice Flour Mix		
Rice flour (1 part)		
Tapioca flour (1 part)		
Cornstarch (1 part)		
Potato flour (1 teaspoon per cup)	3 Tablespoons	4 Tablespoons

Breakfast Food

IDEAS	FOODS and/or recipes in this book
hash browns	Yukon Golds, Russet, Red, Blue/Purple, potatoes O'Brien(peppers & onions)
grains	amaranth, oats?, buckwheat, quinoa, millet, sorghum?
fruit/sweet ingredients	fruit, rosehips(syrup/juice/tea), acerola juice, juice blends
bread & jelly/jam/preserves	(see bread tab), GF sourdough, GF "rye"(caraway, molasses), Udi's breads
breakfast burrito(GF tortilla)	basically the same stuff as omelets--use UDI's GF Tortillas
pancakes	blueberry, banana-nut, mango pancakes, strawberry, etc.
muffins	blueberry, other fruit, banana-nut, etc.
pastries	danishes, puff pastries, baklava(GF phyllo dough??),
proteins	quinoa, tofu/soy, miso, nuts/seeds, supergrain cereal, raspberry-spice granola,
	Nut-free: sunflower seeds, pumpkin seeds, chia, flax, sesame, quinoa, etc.
omelet(egg-free)	onion, peppers, mushroom, tomato, DF cheese or pine nuts
sweeteners	agave, molasses, brown sugar, maple syrup, stevia, date sugar, coconut sugar
milk	hazelnut, soy, coconut, rice, almond, flax, sesame(white & black), etc.
juice	"green" juices, fruit juices, herbal teas, custom-juicing, etc.
combos(protein, starch, carb	hash browns, bread, fruit, nut/soy/sunflower seed butter
	hash browns, pancakes, omelet
	supergrain cereal, hashbrowns, blueberry muffin
	raspberry spice granola, bread, omelet
	burrito, pancakes, hashbrowns
vitamin B supplement	Brewers/Nutritional Yeast (Lewis Labs, etc.)
Note on "dairy free" cheese	Several good "dairy-free" cheeses still have casein (milk protein), however,
	a few do not. (casein is a glue-like substance used for that same purpose)
	Recommendations: Lisanatti almond mozzarella(good taste, texture), casein
	Daiya: mozzarella, cheddar, havarti (dairy-free, casein-free)
	Tofutti cream cheese and sour cream: interesting taste, creamy thick texture
Dairy-free yogurts	Recommendations: So Delicious (coconut milk or almond milk)
Dairy-free ice cream	Recommendations: So Delicious, Turtle Mountain, Almond Dream, etc.

Cakes

1 Black Forest Fruit & Spice Cake
- 20   Medjool dates, pitted
- 20   black mission figs
- 20   black cherries, pitted
- 1/2 c   carob powder
- 1/2 c   chocolate or cocoa/cacao
- 1/4 c   blackstrap molasses, unsulfured
- 1/4 c   coconut, shredded
- 1 c   walnuts, chopped
- 1 tsp   cinnamon
- 1 tsp   cloves
- 1 tsp   allspice
- olive oil for wiping casserole dish/container

Directions: This is a RAW cake, so all that is needed is to blend all ingredients together, and place into oiled 2" casserole dish, and smooth out with a spatula. Using either a spoon and bowl, or an electric mixer, chop and blend together dates, figs, cherries, adding blackstrap molasses gradually. Then add spices, chocolate/cocoa/cacao, and coconut, & blend until smooth. Finally, take walnuts & coat the bottom and sides of dish, scoop out mixture into dish, and evenly sprinkle remaining nuts on top. Chill for up to 2 hours in refrigerator. Serve.

2 Black Forest Cake
Preheat oven to 350. Line 8 or 9 inch springform or cake pan
- 2 c   water (mix w/flaxseed for egg replacer)
- 1 c   flaxseed (egg replacer)
- 1-1/4 c   date sugar/date fines (Chatfield's) or 1-1/4 c brown cane sugar
- 6 Tbsp   corn starch
- 6 Tbsp   brown rice flour | flour mix
- 3/4 c   corn flour
- 3/4 c   sorghum flour
- 3/4 c   carob powder
- 2 c   walnuts, soaked (cream mix)
- 1 c   almonds, soaked
- 16   Brazil nuts
- 1-1/4 c   non-dairy milk beverage (almond, hazelnut, coconut)
- 1/4 c   water w/ 1 tsp sea salt
- 1 or 2   individual vanilla beans, or 2 drops vanilla extract
- 16 oz   black sweet cherries (pitted), with 1/3 c syrup or juice (if not canned, add 1 cup water to cherries after pitting and let sit overnight.

"Kirsch" Sauce
- 2 tsp   cornstarch
- 16 oz   black sweet cherries (pitted)
- 1/4 tsp   apple cider vinegar (preferably with the "mother")
- 1/4 tsp   allspice
- 1/4 tsp   clove powder
- 2 Tbsp   agave nectar, or brown rice syrup

1. Bring saucepan of water to boil, remove from heat. Combine flax mixture and sugar in heatproof bowl or double boiler. Place bowl or pan over pan of water, and beat briskly until mixture leaves a trail. Remove from heat and whisk until cold. Sift flour mixture and carob together, and gently fold into cold mixture with plastic spatula until just combined. Pour into pan and bake for 25 minutes or until cake springs back when pressed.
2. Mix cornstarch with 1/3 of juice from cherries and pour remainder of juice into sauce-

Cakes

(Black Forest Cake continued)
pan. Bring to boil, remove; add in cornstarch and stir until boiling. Remove from heat. Add all cherries except eight (for garnish) to mixture.
3. Puree cherries for Kirsch syrup, then add vinegar, spices and syrup. Blend about 1-2 minutes. Let sit.
4. Use serrated knife to slice cake into 3 layers (or to make it easy, use 3 pans). Spoon some Kirsch syrup over each spoon or pipe cream onto one layer, and add 2nd layer. Spread a thin layer of cream in middle, leaving thick border. Add cherries within border. Cover with 3rd layer. Spread top and sides with cream. Chill 10 minutes. Repeat until desired thickness, and smooth. Garnish each slice with cherry and dust with carob, or press carob chips into side. Refrigerate. Serves 8.
Preparation time: 1.5 - 2 hours plus refrigeration. Total cooking time: 30 minutes.

3   Carrot Spice Marble Cake
Preheat oven to 300 degrees F. Use 8x12x2 pan, or Bundt pan, greased with light olive oil

3 c	medium-large carrots, grated
1/2 c	buckwheat flour
1/2 c	brown rice flour
1/4 c	sorghum flour
1/4 c	amaranth flour
1/2 c	non-dairy milk beverage (soy, almond, hazelnut, coconut, etc.)
1/2 c	orange marmalade
1/2 c	cranberries, fresh, chopped
1 c	walnuts, chopped
1 c	raisins or currants
1 c	flaxseed-water mix (gold or brown flax seed)
1.5 c	olive oil
2 Tbsp	ginger root, freshly grated
1 tsp	lemon juice (unsulfured)
1 tsp	cinnamon
1/2 tsp	cloves powder
1/2 tsp	allspice
1/3 c	pure (Grade AA) dark amber maple syrup
1/4 c	blackstrap molasses (marbling)
2 tsp	sea salt (unrefined)
2 tsp	baking soda

Combine all dry ingredients (flour, spices, sea salt, baking soda), and mix until even-colored. Add liquid or wet ingredients and fruit, flaxseed-water mix, carrots, oil, ginger and maple syrup, and mix until well-blended. Add lemon juice, orange marmalade and nuts, and mix until evenly distributed.
 Use spatula to place mix into well-oiled cake pan (or Bundt pan if desired). Swirl blackstrap molasses around with knife or toothpick for marbling effect. Tap cake pan on countertop to level out batter,and place in oven for 10 minutes, and check to see if cake springs back when pressed. If not,
 bake 5 more minutes and re-check. Cake should be a dark golden-brown, and should spring back when pressed.

Cakes

4 Chocolate Cake (GF-vegan revision)

1.5 c	Bob's Red Mill All-Purpose Gluten-Free baking flour
1 c	date fines (Chatfield's)
1/4 c	cocoa powder, unsweetened
1/4 c	carob powder
1 tsp	baking soda
1 tsp	xanthan gum
3/4 tsp	sea salt
1/2 c	non-dairy milk beverage (soy, nut, rice, nut, coconut)
1/4 c	olive oil or walnut oil
1/4 c	flaxseed-water mixture
1 tsp	vanilla flavoring, or 1 vanilla bean, ground
3/4 c	Butternut (or other DELICIOUS) coffee (warm, 110 degrees F)
1/8 c	peppermint leaves, fresh, coarsely chopped

Preheat oven to 350. Oil 11x7 inch pan with light olive oil. Set aside. Place all ingredients, except coffee, in large bowl and blend with electric mixer. Add coffee and mix until thoroughly blended. Pour into prepared pan and bake for 30-35 minutes or until toothpick comes out clean & cake springs back when pressed. Serves 12

5 Happy Fruit Cake 3.31.2016

1/2 cup	amaranth flour
1/2 cup	buckwheat flour
1/2 cup	brown rice flour
1/8 cup each	sorghum flour, coconut flour, almond flour, quinoa flour
1/4 cup	zante currants
2	plums
2	figs
1	apple
1	pear
1/8 cup	tart cherries
1/8 cup	cranberries
1/8 cup	rosehips
1 Tbsp	orange peel (organic)
2	apricots
1/4 cup	pineapple
1/2 cup	walnuts, chopped
1/4 cup	pistachios
1/2 cup	non-dairy milk (almond milk, etc.)
1 cup	flaxseed-water mix (2:1 water-flaxseed ratio)
1 1/2 cup	olive oil
1 tsp	ginger powder
2 tsp	sea salt
2 tsp	baking soda
2 tsp	org. lemon juice
1 tsp each	cinnamon, cloves, allspice

Use Bundt pan, or 8x12x2 inch pan,

Cakes

6 Tantalizing Torte Chilled Layer Cake   [family dinner dessert]

2 c	hazelnuts/filberts, layer 7 (top)
1 c	raspberries (layer 6)
2 c	raspberry puree (layer 6)
8 oz	baking chocolate, shredded or flaked (layer 5)
2 c	carob powder (layer 4)
1 c	non-dairy milk beverage (layer 4) to add fluffiness to carob powder
1	mango, thinly sliced (layer 3)
1-2 c	coconut, shredded or flaked (layer 2)
1/4 c	organic lemon juice (layer 2)
1/4 c	ginger root, grated (layer 2)
30	Medjool dates, pitted (layer 1--bottom)
1/4 c	pure maple syrup, organic grade A amber, or agave nectar (layer 1--bottom)
1/4 c	blackstrap molasses, unsulphured (layer 1--bottom)
1 tsp	cinnamon (layer 1--bottom)
1 tsp	cloves powder (layer 1--bottom)

Directions: This is a RAW cake, so no cooking/baking required, just mixing and layering ingredients in their appropriate layers. Mix molasses, cinnamon, maple syrup, cloves, and dates. Spread an even layer, about 1/8" thick, of chopped hazelnuts on a sheet of wax paper, in either a springform pan or deep square pan, and scoop 1st layer on top of the nuts. Mix ginger, lemon juice, and coconut, and carefully spread on top of 1st layer. Add mango slices so that they are pointing toward the center of the cake. Whip non-dairy milk beverage (layer 4) with carob powder, to fluffy consistency, and spread over the mango slices. Evenly spread the chocolate flakes over the current layer. Combine the raspberries and raspberry puree, and pour over the chocolate flakes. Finally, sprinkle chopped nuts over the raspberry layer. Best if chilled in refrigerator for at least 2-4 hours, or in freezer for up to 1 hour.

7 Birthday-Cake Black Forest "Bundt-Brownie" with Cherry-Chocolate Sauce 5.21.2014

1 pkg.	Bob's Red Mill GF Brownie Mix

Prepare as directed. Use Bundt pan if desired.

Sauce:

3 oz	GF, dairy-free dark chocolate, 60% + cacao (any flavor), broken into pieces
1 cup	cherries (or 2 cups black cherries), pitted
1 Tbsp	cornstarch
1/2 cup	cold water (combine with cornstarch to make a "slurry"
1/2 cup	brown sugar

Melt chocolate and sugar in thick-walled pan or double boiler over low heat, until melted. Add cornstarch slurry gradually, stirring as you pour. Stir in cherries until coated. Remove from heat and immediately pour over cake for a "chocolate coating".

Cookies, Muffins & Pancakes

1 Blueberry Muffins
Preheat oven to 350

2	ripe bananas
2 c	sorghum flour
2/3 c	Bob's Red Mill Garfava flour
1/2 c	blueberries
1 c	vanilla soymilk (or almond milk)
1/4 c	flaxseed/water mixture
1/8 tsp	xanthan gum
1/8 tsp	sea salt
1 tsp	baking soda
1/2 tsp	pure vanilla flavoring, or 1 vanilla bean

light olive oil for muffin pan (grease with paper towels)

Sift flour into a bowl, and mix in dry ingredients. Blend in remaining ingredients. Fill muffin pan 2/3-3/4 full with mixture, and bake 15-20 minutes until done. Makes 1 dozen muffins.

2 Buckwheat-Blueberry Maple Nut Pancakes

4 cup	buckwheat flour (Arrowhead Mills)
3/4 cup	Bob's Red Mill Gluten-Free All-Purpose baking flour
1 tsp	baking powder
1/2 tsp	baking soda
1/2 tsp	sea salt
2	bananas, mashed
1/2 cup	pure maple syrup
1/2 cup	pecans, coarsely chopped
1/2 cup	blueberries
1/4 cup	flaxseed-water mixture
3/8 cup	molasses, unsulphured
2 tsp	apple cider vinegar
1 tsp	lemon juice
1/4 cup	olive oil
1 tsp	honey to taste

Sift together flour, salt, baking soda and baking powder into a large mixing bowl. In another bowl, whisk together milk, lemon juice, vinegar, flax mixture and oil. Make a hole in the middle of the dry mixture, and pour the liquid mixture into the hole, and mix just until blended. Stir in remainder of ingredients until just combined.

Pour onto hot griddle/flat cooking surface with 1/3 cup measure, and when the edges are bubbly, flip over with a spatula. Wait until the bottom of the pancake is golden brown, then remove the pancake with a spatula to a dish or pan for serving.

Syrup:

1 cup	blueberries
1/3 cup	cold water
2 Tbsp	honey
1/4 tsp	clove powder

Place sauce ingredients into 1-quart sauce pan, over medium heat for about 10 minutes, stirring often to prevent burning.

Cookies, Muffins & Pancakes

3 Carob-Date Confection (my wholesome answer to "donut holes")
- 2 lbs   Medjool dates, pitted
- 1 lb   Turkish organic. apricots (or fresh apricots), unsulphured
- 3/4 tsp   cinnamon
- 1/2 tsp   cloves powder
- 1/2 c   carob powder
- 1/2 c   pure maple syrup, grade A dark amber, or agave nectar
- 1/8 c   blackstrap or organic molasses
- 1 c   walnuts, chopped(coating)
- 1 c   flaxseed, ground(coating)
- 1 c   coconut, shredded (coating)
- 1 c   sesame seed (coating)

(may also use other edible nuts/seeds)
olive oil for rolling (can also refrigerate for 4-12 hours to decrease stickiness)

1 **Split** dates and apricots and remove pit/seed (if necessary). Place dates and apricots into mixer bowl, and using "egg beaters", mix dates and apricots until combined, rotating bowl to evenly mix.

2 Add cinnamon and cloves, maple syrup and carob, mix in for 1-2 minutes. Add molasses, and mix for another 2 minutes.

3 Get 1 small plate for each topping, and put about 1/4 cup of topping onto the plate, refilling as needed. Rub hands with olive oil, and using 2 table spoons (soup size) spoon out about an inch of mixture into one hand, rolling into a 1 inch ball (or 3/4 inch ball to increase quantity), roll completely in desired topping, and set in pan or other container. Repeat process until bowl is scraped clean (for the most part). Makes about 5 dozen decadent, rich balls. Can also squash with fork to make flat cookies. This is a RAW recipe, so there is no need for cooking, as all ingredients are safe to eat as is.

Cookies, Muffins & Pancakes

4 Ginger-Molasses Monster Cookies
- 3/8 cup   flaxseed-water mixture
- 1 tsp   baking powder
- 1 cup   soy, nut, or rice flour
- 1 cup   raisins or currants, moistened in warm water 5 minutes
- 1 cup   buckwheat flour
- 1-1/4 tsp baking soda
- 3/4 cup   yellow corn flour
- 3/4 cup   olive oil
- 1/2 cup   sorghum flour
- 1/2 cup   blackstrap unsulphured molasses
- 1/2 cup   amaranth flour
- 1/4 tsp   sea salt
- 1/4 cup   brown rice flour

Directions: Blend above ingredients and preheat oven to 375 degrees.
- 1/2 cup   cranberries, chopped
- 1/2 cup   applesauce
- 1 tsp   lemon juice
- 1 Tbsp   ginger, ground
- 1/4 tsp   cinnamon,
- 1/4 tsp   cloves
- 1/4 tsp   allspice

Blend into first mixture, and roll into 1-1/2" balls, place on cookie sheet greased with light olive oil or nut oil. Bake at 375 for 10-12 minutes or until toothpick comes out clean. Makes about 3 dozen cookies.

5 Happy Cookies
- 3 Tbsp   flaxseed, chopped (or flaxseed meal)
- 3 Tbsp   apricot preserves, or 3 apricots
- 1 tsp   rosemary
- 1 tsp   mint
- 1 tsp   ginseng
- 1 tsp   fennel seed, chopped
- 1 tsp   apple cider vinegar
- 1 Tbsp   St. John's Wort
- 1 Tbsp   oregano
- 1 Tbsp   Ginkgo biloba
- 1 Tbsp   bee pollen, local (opt.)
- 1 c   water
- 1-1/2 cup sorghum flour, or Bob's GF flour mix
- 1/2 cup   walnuts, chopped
- 1/2 cup   unsulphured blackstrap molasses
- 1/2 cup   organic fresh peanut butter or other nut butter
- 1/4 cup   yellow corn meal
- 1/4 cup   olive oil
- 1/4 cup   buckwheat flour
- 1/8 cup   honey (opt.)
- 1/8 cup   amaranth flour

Combine ingredients, roll into balls, press onto cookie sheet, bake 8-12 minutes at 325.

Cookies, Muffins & Pancakes

6   Maple Pecan Sandies
- 4 c   sorghum flour
- 1 tsp   baking soda
- 3/4 c   soymilk (or other non-dairy milk)
- 1 tsp   lemon juice
- 1 c   olive oil
- 3/8 c   maple syrup, grade A amber
- 3/4 c   pecans, chopped
- 1/8 tsp unrefined sea salt

Combine dry and wet ingredients together, and bake for 8-12 minutes at 325.

7   Mom's Corn Muffins, GF
Preheat oven to 425
- 1/3 c   canola or olive oil
- 1/3 c   brown sugar
- 1   egg, beaten, or 1/4 cup flax-water mixture
- 1-1/4 c soy milk
- 1/2 c   corn flour
- 1/2 c   all-purpose GF flour
- 4 tsp   baking powder
- 1/2 tsp salt
- 1 c   corn meal
- olive oil for greasing muffin pan

Directions: Cream oil and sugar. Add egg(or flax mixture) and milk. Add flour mixed with baking powder and salt. Add corn meal--stir only enough to mix. Grease muffin pans with a paper towel dampened with olive oil. Fill muffin pans 2/3 full. Bake at 425 degrees for 15 minutes. Makes 12-15 muffins.

8   Phil's Chocolate Chip Cookies 2.12.2007 (based on original recipe on Ghirardelli pkg)
1/4 tsp anise seed and 8 whole cloves crushed in mortar & pestle together
1 cup Pillsbury gluten-fre flour
1-1/2 cup Krusteaz GF flour
1 tsp baking soda
1/2 tsp sea salt
2 tsp cinnamon
1/2 cup + 1Tbsp Ghirardelli semi-sweet chocolate chips
1/8 cup Heath toffee bits
1 square Ghirardelli dark chocolate-raspberry, finely chopped
1 ball Lindt white chocolate
1/4 cup chocolate morsels
1/2 cup smart balance butter
1/8 cup olive oil
1/4 cup coconut oil
1/4 cup honey
1 cup brown cane sugar
1/4 cup applesauce, unsweetened
1 egg or 1/4 cup flaxseed-water mix
1/2 tsp vanilla (Madagascar) extract or flavoring

Cookies, Muffins & Pancakes

9 Quinoa Flake Cookies (recipe by Juli Griffith)
- 1 3/4 c   date fines/date sugar
- 1/4 c   carob powder
- 1/4 c   soy or almond (or other vegan) milk
- 1 1/2 c   nut butter (almond, cashew, etc.)
- 3 c   quinoa flakes (or 1.5 cups quinoa flakes, 1.5 cups buckwheat flakes)
- 1 tsp   vanilla extract or pure vanilla flavoring

Combine all ingredients and mix thoroughly. Drop by tablespoonful onto wax paper, let set. Raw recipe. 1 batch makes 4 1/2 dozen cookies.

10 Seven-Layer Bars (Coconut-Pecan Bars) 2018

crust:
coconut flour
millet flour
lemon juice
oatmeal (rolled oats)

Topping:
pecans
coconut-shredded or flaked
brown sugar/creamy substance
butterscotch-type chips

11 Sesame Cookies (Raw)
- 1 cup   brown sesame seeds
- 2 Tbsp   sesame oil, toasted or untoasted
- 2 Tbsp   honey
- 1/4 c   tahini
- 2 Tbsp   fresh ginger

Mix all ingredients and form into balls, or other preferred shape. 'Chill' for 1 hour. Serve.

Desserts, Candy & Pudding

1 Apple-Cinnamon-Caramel Sauce/Syrup   6.1.2014

1 or more	Apple(s) for cooking, sliced thin, or however you like your apples!
1 cup	brown sugar
3 tsp	cinnamon
1 cup	soy or non-dairy milk
1 1/2 tsp	vanilla extract or flavoring

Place apples in a small saucepan, and turn heat on to medium.
Add brown sugar, & stir, until mixture is thick & gooey(about 15 minutes).
Stir continually to prevent mixture from burning on the bottom.
Stir in cinnamon until mixture is desired color. The longer cinnamon is cooked, the more "stringy" it gets, which could be good if you want a gooey sauce! Remove from heat. Can eat either cold or warm, but best eaten warm! Delicious! If you want "milk" in your caramel, coconut, almond or hazelnut milks would be most appropriate as these are primarily "dessert" nut milks.

For a chocolate alternative, I like to use the "heavy-duty" Dairy-Free chocolate bars, as in, 60% or better cacao content. For this you may need a "double boiler", or putting a bowl or other pan inside the pan on the burner, to (yes) prevent burning. Do not fill the pan on the burner more than half-full of water, otherwise, the water will spill out. After filling the pan with water (1 inch), put the top bowl or pan in, and any excess water will come out (preferably do this over the sink, not the stove). Melting the chocolate will take awhile, so stir every few minutes, and when you see chocolate getting liquid-y, add your other ingredients, and stir until the mixture is a thick liquid. Overheating hardens chocolate! You can use these sauces/syrups on cinnamon rolls, vegetable crudités, popcorn(?), cakes, or anything that would be better with caramel or chocolate!

2 Baklava (GF, Raw rev.)

3-1/2 oz	walnuts, chopped for filling
8 oz	organic raw honey
10 oz	fig preserves (St. Dalfour Royal Fig Spread), or Turkish figs
1-3/4 lb	Medjool dates, pitted
3-1/2 oz	walnuts, finely chopped (coating)
Directions:	If using dried figs, let soak in warm water for 30 minutes. Lay out half of pitted dates (skin down) over half of finely chopped walnuts on sheet of wax paper in a 9x13 casserole dish. Press dates to flatten, or use roller. Mix honey, fig preserves, and chopped walnuts, and spread over bottom date mixture. Produce another "date cover" with remaining half of dates, coat date skins with remainder of walnut fines, and invert so that the date skins are on top. Press down around the edges to seal, and remove all wax paper. Makes a gooey, exotic delicacy without messing around with phyllo dough. Cut into 2"-3" triangles for serving, if desired. Total prep time: ~ 2 hours

Desserts, Candy & Pudding

3 Chocolate Pizza (Dark Chocolate) 12.24.2015 made for family dinner

1-3 5 oz bars	dark chocolate (non-dairy) mint
2 tsp	organic vanilla flavoring
3/4 cup	raw org. cacao
1 1/2 cup	shredded coconut
1 cup	Thai Kitchen coconut milk
1 1/4 cup	soy milk
1/3 cup	dried tart chierries
1/2 cup	Hershey's (or other brand) semi sweet chocolate chips
7	raspberries, chopped
1/2 cup	dried cranberries

Note: orange & coconut garnish on no-nuts section.   Pecans, hazelnuts & pistachios on nut section

1 Tbsp	crushed organic red rose petals (Frontier Herbs & Spices, or at your local organic co-op)

Directions: Using a 15-inch shallow (1/2") pizza pan for the container, wipe some olive oil on the pan. Use a double-boiler pan set-up to melt the chocolate, chips and cacao on MED-LOW heat, stirring occasionally until completely melted. Slowly add coconut milk, soy milk & vanilla, stir in to chocolate mixture. Reduce heat to low, to keep liquefied, and cut some wax paper to fit the pan for pouring the liquid chocolate into the pan for cooling. Prepare the remainder of the ingredients.
Pour the liquid chocolate into the pizza pan with the wax paper and let cool and solidify. Decorate the chocolate while still warm with the remaining ingredients.

4 Carobbean Fruit Parfait

3 c	non-dairy yogurt, or "nut cream" (soaked and pureed almonds, cashews, etc.)
1/8 c	carob powder
1 c	blueberries
1 c	raspberries
1	mango, diced 1/2"
1	kiwifruit, sliced and skinned, 1/4" thick(should get 8 slices)
1 c	banana, sliced 1/4"
1/8 c	peppermint leaves, fresh, chopped
1 sprig	mint for garnish (3 leaves)
6	macadamia nuts, whole, raw, unsalted

Stir 1 Tbsp carob and mint into yogurt until thoroughly mixed. Spoon 1/2 cup of mixture into bottom of glass. Layer 1/2 cup of diced mango on top. Layer next with 1/2 cup yogurt, 1/2 cup bananas, blueberries,1/2 cup raspberries, followed by 1/2 cup yogurt. Place 4 slices of kiwifruit in a square (1 slice each for the top,2 sides and bottom). Place macadamia nuts as points in an equilateral triangle. Garnish with the mint sprig in the center, and serve.

5 Cookies & Cream Pudding idea   2017/18
cashew with macadami cream, carob powder/cocoa flecks, baking chocolate, vanilla bean

Desserts, Candy & Pudding

6 Mulled Blueberry Pudding
- 1 qt — blueberries, fresh or frozen
- 1 tsp — cinnamon
- 1 tsp — cloves
- 1 tsp — allspice
- 1/4 c — pure maple syrup, grade A

Directions: Place blueberries into blender, and puree, adding water as needed to remain liquid. Add spices, reduce speed and add maple syrup, and mix until thick but still smooth and creamy.

Note: For large batches (1 or more dozen people), adding 1/2 tsp xanthan gum may be recommended for thickening(evenly divided between batches).

7 Pistachio Pudding
- 4 c — pistachios, fresh, raw, shelled
- 1/4 c — peppermint leaves, fresh, coarsely chopped
- 2 c — walnuts, coarsely chopped
- 1 c — pineapple, dehydrated & unsulphured, chopped (1/4")
- 2 c — macadamia nuts, creamed, or macadamia nut butter
- 1 c — cashews, raw or lightly roasted, creamed, or cashew butter or cashew milk

Blend with mixer until smooth and creamy.
Makes about 2 1/2 quarts of pudding (5/8 gallon)

Note: Chopping nuts in the blender or using a blender to "milk" the nuts produces a gritty, unappetizing texture to the pudding.

8 Rhubarb Fruit Crisp   Vegan, Gluten-free   9.12.2013 **Use 9"x9"x2" casserole dish

Crust:
- 1/3 cup — Bob's Red Mill GF All-Purpose Flour
- 1/3 cup — Bob's Red Mill Organic. Quinoa Flour
- 1/3 cup — Arrowhead Mills Buckwheat Flour

Topping:
- 1 cup — Quaker Oats Quick-oats
- 2 Tbsp — cinnamon
- 1/2 cup — Smart Balance (60%~ vegetable oil spread), or use Coconut Oil
- 1 cup — brown sugar
- 1/2 cup — English walnuts, chopped (or may use sunflower seeds or pumpkin seeds)

Filling:
- 15 oz or 1 lb — peaches, sliced
- 12 oz — apricot pie filling, or use fresh apricots
- 1 cup — rhubarb stalk, 1/4" sliced
- 1 cup — cherries, pitted

Sift and combine all flours into a bowl, mix, add cold water and knead until dough is firm enough to form a solid ball. Dust a breadboard or cutting board with flour (GF), divide dough into 2 even halves, and work both into a flat square 12" x 12". Carefully peel dough off of board and drape over casserole dish so dough is centered. Cut off any extra, and fit dough into container. Melt butter-spread, combine topping ingredients, stir until evenly mixed, and set aside. Combine filling ingredients and stir together until evenly

3 mixed. Pour into casserole dish on top of bottom crust. Drape top crust over dish, and crimp edges of crust to seal. Spread topping evenly over top crust.

4 Bake at 350 degrees for 20-30 minutes, until topping & crust is golden brown.

Crust mix makes 3 cups -- use 1 1/2 cups on bottom, 1 1/2 cups on top

Desserts, Candy & Pudding

9 Gourmet Rice Krispie Bars   1.7.2017 idea
- Rice Krispies cereal
- macadamia nut butter
- almond butter
- pistachios
- coconut-agave
- raw cacao
- Italian: arborio rice & pine nuts

10 Rosehip Syrup

vitamin C, soak rose hips in room temp water 30 minutes to soften for eating, makes delicious healthy syrup. Recommendation: obtain hips from either Frontier Herbs, or grow an organic Rosa canina bush, which is a primary source of these medicinal rosehips.

11 Streudel for 4 hotel full-pans of fruit cobbler/crisp (done at Sheraton)

1-1/2 quarts	flour
1 pound	butter
4 cups	brown sugar
3 Tbsp	cinnamon
1 tsp	nutmeg
2 Tbsp	cloves

Makes 3 quarts
Dice butter into /2 inch wide pieces, mix into flour until butter is about pea-size.
Add brown sugar to flour mixture and mix in.
Add spices and mix in. (when you get the spice mixture like you want, you can make it ahead of time, and add more to taste)
Note: All mixing should be done with both hands in order to get butter to pea size (for flakiness)
Bake uncovered for 30 minutes at 325 F, until golden brown.

12 Sweet Peach Chutney

3/4 c	date sugar, as syrup in room temperature water (70 degrees. F)
1/8 tsp	pure vanilla
1/8 tsp	cinnamon
1/8 tsp	cloves powder
2 c	peaches, fresh preferred (frozen okay, let thaw)
1/2 c	dates
1/4 c	pistachios
1/4 c	walnuts
3 c	apricots, fresh
1/2 c	date sugar, dry (brown sugar, turbinado, or coconut sugar if date not available)
1/2 cup	red bell pepper
1 Tbsp	ginger root

Combine dates, apricots, peaches & vanilla in 6-quart pan, heat on medium until warm (100 degrees). Combine pepper, ginger, date sugar, cloves & cinnamon, allow to marinate until apricot mixture is done. Add chutney mix and half of nuts to apricot mixture, stir to blend, garnish with remaining nuts.

Desserts, Candy & Pudding

13 Whipped Topping - natural (idea) 9.23.2004
    nut oil
    coconut finely shred
    soaked nuts
    coconut oil/milk
    pure vanilla

14 Wild Rice Pudding PSK 1.7.16 (idea--instead of boring white rice pudding)

1 Eggless Cornbread Quiche
- 12 oz   polenta (2 tubes), traditional polenta, or gluten-free cornbread mix
- 2/3 c   non-dairy milk
- 2 Tbsp   Italian seasoning, or other seasoning, to taste
- 1 c   vegetable filling (spinach, carrots, parsley, etc.)

Directions: Cook polenta in skillet, and blend in remaining ingredients in last half of cooking time. Allow to cook until golden brown on bottom, then flip over, and cook until "bottom" is golden brown. Flip over again if desired, and serve. *Note: use a pizza pan to help flip it over if needed.

Parmesan Cheese
- pine nuts, minced
- (see also "Breakfast Foods" for more on cheese)

Breakfast Sausage Blend
- buckwheat groats
- sage
- black pepper
- thyme
- coriander
- fennel seed

Pasta & Pizza

1 Borscht Lasagna   12/22/2014
1 pkg.	Tinkyada rice lasagna noodles (12 noodles)
1	beet, grated
3	carrots, grated
2 quarts	marinara or pasta sauce
1/2 cup	red onion, diced
1 cup	dry garbanzo beans, cooked — cook these together
1/8 cup	millet, cooked — first for 30 minutes
1	zucchini, sliced
4 oz	[marinated] artichoke hearts
2	red bell peppers, halved and julienned
1/4 cup	quinoa flakes
1/4 cup	buckwheat flour
1/4 cup	flaxseed meal
2 Tbsp	Italian seasoning
4	garlic cloves, sliced
1/2 cup	Italian parsley leaves
1 tsp	cumin
1/2 cup	olive oil plus enough to grease the casserole dish

Directions:
Oil 9x15x2 casserole dish with olive oil & paper towel. Combine marinara sauce with carrots, artichokes, beet, buckwheat flour, flax, garlic, cumin, parsley, olive oil, onion & Italian seasoning. Stir together. Pour 1/2 cup of sauce into casserole, place 3 noodles on top, then a layer of zucchini, sauce, noodles, a layer of peppers, 3 more noodles, sauce, 3 more noodles, garbanzo beans and millet, 3 more noodles, and the last of the sauce, and place the remainder of the red peppers. Cover dish with foil, and bake at 350 degrees for 40 minutes to 1 hour. Serves about 12. Approximately 2 hours prep time.

2 GF Vegan Vegetable Lasagna   Preheat oven to bake at 300 degrees.
15	rice lasagna noodles, Tinkyada or equivalent (need 4" deep 9x13 lasagna pan)
60 oz	marinara or chunky garden pasta sauce
3	medium carrots, grated
2	medium zucchini, sliced
2	red or yellow bell peppers, halved and sliced
8 oz	spinach, fresh, stems removed
8	porcini or button mushrooms, sliced 1/8", OR
1	Portabello mushroom, halved and sliced 1/4"
2 c	artichoke hearts
1/8 cup	Italian seasoning, or fresh versions of rosemary, basil, oregano, thyme, marjoram
1 c	Italian parsley, fresh, coarsely chopped
1 Tbsp	cumin, ground
1 Tbsp	coriander
1 Tbsp	lemon-pepper, salt-free
1 c	pine nuts, finely chopped
	extra-virgin olive oil

Directions Combine pasta sauce with herbs & spices, & 1/2 cup olive oil. Cook noodles 7-10 minutes(al dente), with 1/4 cup olive oil. Layer 1 1/4 cups sauce on bottom of pan under 1st layer of noodles. Top with carrots, sauce & 2nd layer of noodles, mushrooms, sauce, & 3rd layer of noodles, with spinach, sauce, & 4th layer of noodles, then artichokes, sauce, & 5th layer of noodles. Final layer: red peppers, sauce, sprinkle with pine nuts. Bake for 30 minutes.

Pasta & Pizza

3 Linguine Alfredo Primavera   6.7.2014

1 pkg.	linguine noodles
1	zucchini, sliced
1	red bell pepper, julienne
3	common mushrooms, sliced
1	carrot, bias-sliced
5 leaves	fresh basil, torn---sauté vegetables in olive oil over medium heat 3-5 minutes until al dente (chewy but not crunchy)

Sauce

6 oz total	cream & butter (may increase cream, or use vegan butter)
1 Tbsp	fresh rosemary
1/4 cup	white onion, diced
1/4 cup	corn starch slurry(1 Tbsp:1/4 cup cool water)

Sauté onions and some minced garlic in olive oil for 5 minutes on medium, then stir in cream & butter, and rosemary. Cook for about 5-10 minutes until thick. Stir in corn starch slurry until sauce is desired thickness.
Place pasta on a plate, top with vegetable mixture, serve.

4 Pasta Primavera

1-1/2 cups	pasta of choice, or zested vegetable pasta (zucchini, sweet potato, carrot)
1/2 c	broccoli florets
8 spears	asparagus, cut in 1" pieces
4	artichoke hearts
1	carrot, sliced
1/3 cup	garbanzo beans or cannellini beans, dry
2	garlic cloves, minced
1/2 cup	pine nuts, pureed
1/4 cup	extra virgin olive oil, pureed with pine nuts (oil should be pre-chilled)
1 sprig	parsley, fresh
1 sprig	rosemary, fresh
3 leaves	basil, fresh

Cook garbanzo beans for 30 minutes. Prepare vegetables, and cook pasta if necessary. Drain pasta, and combine with vegetables, adding garbanzo beans and fresh herbs for garnish. Top with pine nut mixture and serve.

5 Phil's Pasta Salad (for Sheraton event) 2.20.2016

10 lbs	cooked pasta
2 Tbsp	minced garlic
1/4 cup	olive oil
1/4 cup	mayonnaise & heavy cream
1 Tbsp	red wine vinegar
1 Tbsp	dried basil
1 Tbsp	dried oregano
1 Tbsp	dried rosemary (cooked in water 30 seconds, let sit for 10 minutes to plump up)
1 tsp	garlic powder
2	zucchini, quartered, 1/4"
2	cucumbers, peeled, sliced in 6ths lengthwise and sliced 1/4" across
5	4" celery sticks, minced
1 cup	shredded carrots, chopped
1 cup	red cabbage, chopped
1 cup each	red and green bell peppers
1/4 cup	red onion, minced

6 Penne Garden Pasta Salad

16 oz	Tinkyada brown rice penne pasta
25-1/2 oz	garden vegetable spaghetti sauce
1/2 oz	dried Portabello mushrooms
5 oz	baby spinach
1 cup	garbanzo beans, dried (or 15oz can)
2	carrots, grated
1	red onion, diced
2	garlic cloves, sliced
2 tsp	Italian seasoning
2 Tbsp	extra virgin olive oil

Soak dried Portabello mushrooms for 30 minutes in warm water. Cook penne according to directions with 1 Tbsp oil. Combine sauce, garlic & Italian seasoning, warm over low heat 10 minutes. Combine vegetables and garbanzo beans with mushrooms, place on top of pasta, or mix into pasta. Pour sauce over mixture and serve.

7 Quinoa Alfredo Primavera

varies	white, red or black quinoa, or quinoa pasta--cook according to directions
1	chayote squash, boiled 10-15 minutes until tender
1	red bell pepper, 1" julienne, or diced chili pepper
1/2 cup	red onion or Spanish onion, 1/4" dice
1	avocado, sliced
1/4 cup	olive oil
1/4 cup	coconut cream, to taste
1/4 cup	cilantro, fresh
1 tsp	cumin

Cook quinoa 7-10 minutes, and cook chayote squash. Mix quinoa with onion, olive oil, coconut cream and cumin. Top with pepper, onion, cilantro & sliced avocado. Serve.

8 Quinoa Pasta Salad

1 lb	quinoa pagoda pasta
1 c	Spanish, or red onion, sliced 1/4"
1 c	tomato, diced 3/8"
1	avocado, sliced 1/8"
1	jalapeno, minced
2 Tbsp	parsley leaves, fresh
2	garlic cloves, minced
1/2 tsp	cumin
1 Tbsp	cilantro
1 sprig	cilantro (garnish)
1/2 cup	olives (garnish)
1 sprig	parsley, fresh
1 sprig	rosemary, fresh
3 leaves	basil, fresh
1/4 c	extra virgin olive oil, pureed w/pine nuts (oil should be chilled)
extra	extra virgin olive oil

Cook pasta for 8-10 minutes until al dente. Drain, and toss with olive oil. Combine tomato, jalapeno, garlic, onion, dry cumin, parsley & cilantro. Using blender or food processor, puree pine nuts, add oil, blend 2 minutes.
Mix pasta with vegetable mixture, top with pine nuts, olives and fresh herbs.

Pasta & Pizza

9 Spelt Pizza (non-wheat/vegan revision from <u>The Classic Italian Cookbook</u> (J. della Croce)

1 envelope	dry yeast
3-1/2 oz	warm water (70-80 degrees)
4 c	whole grain spelt flour, plus flour for dusting (additional cup)
1-1/2 tsp	sea salt
7 oz	cold water
2 Tbsp	olive oil, plus extra for brushing
1 Tbsp	pizza seasoning
2 pkgs.	soy or almond cheese ('**Lisanatti**' is highly recommended), mozzarella style, or **Daiya**
2 Tbsp	olive oil for dough glaze
1 Tbsp	pizza seasoning w/o bell peppers for dough glaze
3 Tbsp	pizza seasoning for sauce (to taste)
1 Tbsp	fennel seed
15 oz	tomato puree
1 Tbsp	extra-virgin olive oil for sauce
2 Tbsp	artichoke or olive tapenade

Pizza Crust Directions:
Combine yeast and one-half of the warm water, and let stand in a warm place for 10 minutes, or until mixture is foamy. Sift together 1 cup of the flour, and the salt, then make a well in the middle of the flour. Add the rest of the warm water, plus the cold water, and oil to the yeast mixture, then pour this liquid into the well. Slowly stir the flour into the liquid until it is absorbed. Sift in another 2 cups of the flour. When dough becomes too stiff to stir, shape it into a ball.
Transfer dough to floured board, and knead for 8-10 minutes until silky and elastic, adding flour as needed. Place dough in lightly oiled bowl, and brush with oil. Cover bowl and let rise for 1-2 hours at room temperature, until doubled in size.
Punch dough to expel the air, then oil a baking sheet or preheat a baking stone.
Knead dough until elastic, then cut into number of desired sections if making more than one pizza. Flatten dough into a disk with your hands, and stretch it, working outwards from the center. Transfer to baking sheet, cover with clean towels and let rise for 30 minutes.

Toppings:
Brush pizza base with oil, place toppings on pizza, glaze crust with Pizza seasoning and oil.
Thin crust 14 inch=7 minutes, 8 inch crusts=3-4 minutes. 1/4 inch crust: 6"=4 minutes,12"=9 min.
1/2" (focaccia base) crust + 10-11 minutes. Bake at 400 degrees for time listed for your pizza size.

Pasta & Pizza

10 Traditional Lasagna   need: 4" deep lasagna pan, 9x15
- 15   lasagna noodles
- 2 qts   marinara or garden vegetable pasta sauce
- 2 c   buckwheat groats, marinated in coriander, fennel seed, sage & black pepper
- 1   red bell pepper, halved, julienne
- 1   medium carrot, grated
- 1   medium zucchini, sliced
- 4   mushrooms (button, porcini) fresh, sliced
- 1 c   Italian parsley
- 2   garlic cloves, minced
- 1/4 c   Italian seasoning
- 1 Tbsp   coriander
- 1 Tbsp   cumin
- 2 pkgs. soy or almond mozzarella-style cheese ('Lisanatti') for topping
- 3/4 c   extra virgin olive oil--1/4 cup for noodles, 1/2 cup for sauce

Combine marinara or pasta sauce, cumin, coriander, Italian seasoning, garlic, 1/2 cup olive oil & Italian parsley. Cook noodles according to directions. Combine 1 1/2 cups buckwheat groats, 3 2/3 Tbsp coriander, 2 Tbsp fennel seed, 2 Tbsp sage, and 1 tsp black pepper, in 3 cups water, and simmer over medium heat for 10 minutes or until noodles are done.
Combine buckwheat mixture with sauce, and layer 10 2/3 oz (1 1/3 cups) sauce mixture on bottom of pan, lay 3 noodles side by side with 1/4" between. Top with carrots, and 2nd layer of sauce. Add 2nd layer of noodles, zucchini and sauce. Add 3rd layer of noodles, mushrooms and sauce. Add 4th layer of noodles, red peppers and sauce. Add 5th layer of noodles, last of sauce, and top evenly with vegan cheese.
Bake in 400 degree oven for 30-50 minutes or until cheese is golden brown.

other pasta ideas: raw vegetable pasta (saladacco, other tools), raw ravioli or cannoli

Pies & Tarts

1 GF Chocolate Pie (GF revision from **The Dessert Bible**,p.253,C. Kimball) 1/3/2015

- 1 fully prebaked 9-inch Mi-Del Gluten-free graham pie crust

Filling: *(coconut milk is used in place of heavy cream(dairy) in the original recipe)*

- 9 oz semisweet and/or bittersweet chocolate, chopped
- 4 1/8 Tbsp butter (can use "Smart Balance", or other spreadable vegetable oil, etc.)
- 3/4 cup Thai Kitchen regular coconut milk (may need to stir to incorporate)

Melt chocolate and butter over low heat in either a heavy pan or double-boiler, stirring occasionally, until just melted. Remove from heat and add coconut cream, stir until mixture is smooth. If necessary, place mixture back on heat to smooth out the mixture. Pour mixture into pie shell (this will fill up to within 3/8 to 1/2 inch of the crust rim) and cool (place in refrigerator) until ready to serve.

2 Pecan Pie

- 12 large dates (Medjool, etc.) for crust
- 12 almonds, walnuts or pecans (crust)
- 2-3 cups pecans for filling, chopped
- 1 c brown flaxseed mixture (filling)
- 1/4 c pure maple syrup (filling)
- 1-2 c cashews, almonds, or macadamias, (whipped topping)
- water for cream
- 1/2 cup pecan halves (garnish)

Mix dates and nuts for crust. Press into pie pan and smooth out.
Combine flaxseed, maple syrup and pecans for filling.
Scoop filling mixture into crust. Bake for 10 minutes at 200 to warm up.
Garnish with remaining pecans. Serve.

3 Turtle Pie

Crust:
- 4 cups pecan pieces, chopped
- 4 cups almonds, chopped
- 2/3 cup blackstrap molasses, unsulphured

Mix above until evenly coated
- 2/3 cup high-fat cocoa powder for bottom of pan

Caramel Sauce: (recipe from Connor Roche, Sheraton)
- 4 cups brown sugar
- 1/2 Cup Thai Kitchen coconut milk or equivalent
- 4 Tbsp coconut oil or vegan butter (originally butter)
- pinch sea salt
- 1 Tbsp PURE vanilla extract (or flavoring)

Mix sugar, cream, oil & salt in saucepan over medium-low heat. Cook while whisking gently for 5-7 minutes until contents are melted and blended. Add vanilla & cook 1 more minute.

Cheesecake:
[get creative]

Pickles, Relish, Salsa & Sauce

1 Black Bean and Corn Relish
- 3 lb black beans, cooked or soaked until tender
- 48 oz yellow corn kernels (frozen), thawed
- 1 cup red onion, chopped
- 1 jalapeno pepper, minced
- 2 garlic cloves, minced
- 2 green onions, sliced 1/4"
- 10 sprigs cilantro, coarsely chopped
- 1 Tbsp chili powder
- 1 Tbsp cumin
- 2 cups red or yellow bell pepper, or pimentos, chopped
- 1/2 cup Spanish extra virgin olive oil
-   lime juice, to taste

2 Afterburner Untomato Salsa
- 2 Jalapeno peppers
- 1 Poblano pepper
- 1 Habanero pepper
- 4 mild red chilies (Fresno, etc.)
- 1 Serrano pepper
- 1/4 cup Spanish onion
- 1/4 cup Red onion
- 1/4 cup cilantro, fresh
- 4 garlic cloves
- 1 Tbsp basil, fresh

Rinse and mince chili peppers. Mince red onion, cilantro, garlic and basil. Combine peppers, onions and herbs.

3 Chili Verde Salsa
- 1 Poblano pepper, green
- 1 Anaheim pepper, green
- 1 Jalapeno peppers, green
- 1 Serrano pepper, green
- 1 green onions
- 1 tomatillo
- 1 avocado
- 1/4 cup epazote (if available)
- 1/2 cup cilantro
- 1 Tbsp apple cider vinegar

4 Coconut Milk Sauce 6.5.2014
- 13 oz can Thai Kitchen coconut milk, original
- 1/2 tsp ginger root
- 1 cup peanuts, dry roasted, unsalted (or cashews, etc.)
- 1 tsp lemon grass
- 1 Tbsp sesame seed
- 1/2 tsp garlic, minced

5 Medium Salsa
- 1 c   Poblano pepper, diced
- 1   jalapeno, minced
- 2   large or Roma tomatoes, diced
- 1/4 c jicama, diced
- 1/4 c Spanish onion, diced
- 1   garlic clove, minced
- 1 Tbsp cilantro, fresh, minced
- 1 Tbsp juice of a lime

6 Medium Untomato Salsa
- 1   jalapeno, minced
- 1/2 c Poblano pepper
- 1/8 c Spanish onion
- 1/8 c Red onion
- 3   mild red chilies (Fresno, etc.)
- 1   garlic clove
- 1/8 cup cilantro leaves
- 1 Tbsp juice of a lime

7 Mom's Amazing Zucchini Relish
- 12 c   zucchini, sliced
- 4 c   white onion, sliced
- 5 Tbsp sea salt

Put in bowl, let set at room temperature overnight. In morning, wash thoroughly with cold water, & grind in food mill(crank style) with one green or yellow pepper and 1 red pepper. Combine and cook.

- 1   red bell pepper, sliced
- 1   yellow bell pepper, sliced
- 2-1/2 c apple cider vinegar
- 2 c   honey
- 1 Tbsp dry mustard
- 1 Tbsp cornstarch
- 3/4 tsp turmeric
- 1-1/2 tsp celery seed
- 1/2 tsp white pepper

Combine in pan and simmer 30 minutes. Put in jar or plastic container with lid. Makes 5 pints.

8 Pesto
- 8 parts fresh basil (or any other leafy herb)
- 4 parts olive oil
- 2 parts walnuts and/or pine nuts
- 1 part lemon juice

9 Pesto Cream Sauce with almond milk 9.1.2015
- fresh basil (or other herbs)
- garlic
- pine nuts
- extra-virgin olive oil
- almond milk
- coconut flour

Mix above ingredients together and let marinate.

Pickles, Relish, Salsa & Sauce

10 Pickles (cucumber, non-alum)
- 5-10 small cucumbers
- 1/2 c raw apple cider vinegar (Bragg)
- 1 Tbsp dill weed
- 3 garlic cloves
- 1 Tbsp peppercorns
- pickling spices (if desired)

11 Pickled Red Onions & Cucumbers
- 1 onion, red or white, sliced
- 1 medium cucumber, sliced
- 1/2 cup apple cider vinegar
- 1 Tbsp dill weed
- 1 Tbsp dill seed
- 1 garlic clove, minced
- 1 tsp parsley, minced
- 1 tsp caraway seeds
- 1 tsp Celtic sea salt, coarse (may also use Mediterranean sea salt)
- 1/4 cup red radish, sliced
- 1/4 cup jicama, diced (or turnip, kohlrabi, etc.)
- 1/4 cup fennel stalk, chopped

Combine ingredients in a large (stainless steel) bowl and mix together. Refrigerate for at least 5-7 days to allow for marinating.

12 Pico de Gallo
- 1/4 cup Jicama, small dice
- 1 large tomato, diced
- 1 jalapeno, diced
- 1/4 cup Spanish onion, diced
- 2 tomatillos, diced
- 2 stalks green onion, sliced
- 1/4 cup cilantro, coarsely chopped
- 1 Tbsp juice of a lime

13 Salsa Blanca
- 1/2 cup Jicama
- 1 banana pepper or Hungarian wax pepper
- 1 Tbsp horseradish root
- 1/4 cup coconut milk
- 1/4 cup soaked white quinoa
- 4 Brazil nuts, skin removed, soaked & creamed
- 1/8 cup Spanish onion, finely chopped
- 2 garlic cloves, finely minced
- 1/4 cup soaked amaranth seed
- 1 tsp white pepper

Pickles, Relish, Salsa & Sauce

14 Super Hot Sauce
- 2 c   barbeque sauce
- 1/2 c   red-pepper sauce
- 1/2 c   tabasco sauce
- 5 Tbsp   habanero pepper sauce
- 1/4 c   honey
- 4 Tbsp   red pepper flakes
- 2 Tbsp   black pepper
- 2 Tbsp   cayenne pepper
- 4 tsp   basil leaves

Mix together all ingredients. No need to cook. Let sit for 30 minutes to blend flavors. Actually tested on customers (buffalo wing sauce).

15 Souped-up Black Bean & Corn Relish   7/13/2014 (made for Solar Club picnic)   MILD
- 1 can   black beans
- 1 can   chili beans
- 10 oz   yellow corn
- 1 Tbsp   ginger root, grated
- half   jicama
- 1   jalapeno
- 1   red bell pepper
- 1   red onion
- 2   tomatillo
- 1   chayote squash
- 1   whole fresh lime w/juice, squeezed & thinly sliced
- 1   avocado
- 1 tsp   chili powder
- 10 sprigs cilantro
- ~1/4 cup   extra virgin olive oil

Salads & Dressings

1 Ambrosia Salad

1 cup	strawberries, fresh
1	bananas, fresh, sliced
1 cup	coconut, fresh, shredded or flaked
1/4 cup	agave nectar
1/4 cup	date sugar (opt.)

Puree strawberries in blender for 1 minute.
Combine pureed strawberries and remaining ingredients into a bowl and mix until evenly-blended. Serve cool.

2 Asian Dish 6.29.2015

5	parsnips, halved & sliced
2	Fresno peppers
5 fresh	shiitake mushrooms
1	Daikon radish
1	red bell pepper
1/3 cup	sesame seed
1 cup	tahini
1/8 cup (full)	ginger root, large-grated
1.5 cups	snow peas, halved
4 leaves	mustard greens
1/4 cup	toasted sesame oil
1 Tbsp	5-spice powder
8 oz	mandarin oranges
1	carrots, sliced on bias
1/8 cup	lemon grass, 1/8" slice
1/2 cup	red onion, 3/8" dice
1/4 cup	coconut oil
1/4 cup	Bragg liquid aminos
1/4 cup	olive oil

3 Asian Salad/Slaw

1 head	Napa Chinese Cabbage, 1/2 inch strips {or Bok Choy for a distinct taste}
1	large carrot, match stick cut, 1-1/2" x 1/8"
1/4 cup	ginger root, finely grated
1/2 cup	cilantro, fresh, lightly chopped
1	large red bell pepper, halved, and 1/4 inch julienne strips
8 oz	Mung bean sprouts [for fresh, you need 3-5 days for the sprouting process]
1/4 cup	brown sesame seed
1 cup dry	garbanzo beans, adzuki or soy beans
8 oz	Bragg's Liquid Aminos pure soy sauce
2 stalks	lemon grass, sliced, with 1/2 inch of each end cut off and discarded
6 oz fresh	shiitake mushrooms(or 1/2 oz dry)
1/2 cup	red onion, diced 1/4 inch
6 oz	sesame oil, or to taste
3 Tbsp	5-spice powder (see *Seasonings*)
	or (ingredients below)
2 pods	star anise (star pod with seeds)
2 Tbsp	fennel seed
1 Tbsp	cinnamon
1 Tbsp	clove powder
1 tsp	white pepper

Salads & Dressings

Asian Salad/Slaw cont'd

Directions: Puree 5-spice powder, lemongrass and shiitake mushrooms together until smooth.*** Hand-mix this sauce with the oil. For emulsion, mix in blender. Rinse cabbage leaves under running water, gently shake off excess water. Tip: Because this recipe makes about 1-1/2 gallons of salad, put Napa cabbage into 1 large bowl, and put remainder of mixture into another large bowl, and mix the remainder of ingredients, then evenly mix the cabbage and the mixture into 1 bowl, or 2x9x13 inch pans, and put the combined mixture of the soy sauce, blended sauce and oil into a 4-cup measuring cup with spout, mix with whisk, and pour 1/2 of this mixture evenly over each container of salad. Combine contents of both bowls as individual servings, or mix together in one bowl and store in refrigerator. Get ready for a healthy taste sensation!

*** **Note for sauce: may need to use some Liquid Aminos to puree the ingredients.**

4   **Asian Salad-Indian Version 2/28/2015 (H.I.S. banquet)**
   mustard greens
   Napa cabbage
   Bragg liquid aminos
   untoasted sesame oil
   adzuki beans
   red bell pepper
   shishito pepper
   shallot
   garlic
   sesame seed
   goji berries
   shiitake mushrooms
   cardamom powder
   5-spice powder
   ginger root
   cilantro
   lemongrass
   carrot
   red onion

5   **Beans-n-Greens Salad 6.10.2017**
   light red kidney beans
   great northern beans
   broccoli
   sunflower seeds
   carrot
   romaine
   power greens (kale, spinach, chard)
   avocado
   radish-clover sprouts
   Italian seasoning
   olive oil
   Bragg's Liquid Aminos
   lemon pepper seasoning (grinder)

Salads & Dressings

6   Curried Bean Salad 6.17.2017

        tri-beans (kidney, pinto, black)
        garbanzo beans
        fresh dill
        2 carrots
        parsnip
        green leaf lettuce
        red onion
        snow peas, de-stemmed
        avocado, sliced
        sunflower seeds
        olive oil
        liquid aminos
        ginger, grated fresh
        red radish
        flaxseed meal
        lime juice
        fresh thyme
        cucumber, quartered
        pumpkin curry sauce (Special Selection, Kroger)
        pistachio meats, raw, unsalted

7   4-Pepper Mexican Salad 3.21.16

1/3 cup	olive oil
1	jicama, diced
1	tomatillo, diced
3	crimini mushrooms, sliced
2	carrots, sliced
1/3 cup	red cabbage, sliced
1 3rd	red bell pepper, julienne
1	jalapeno, minced
1	Thai chili pepper, minced
1	Anaheim pepper, minced
1	avocado, diced
1	10-oz bag org. yellow frozen corn kernels
1	zucchini, diced
2	15-oz cans chili beans
2	garlic, minced
3/4" slice	red onion, diced
1/4 cup	dry garbanzos, cooked
1/8 cup	sprouted quinoa mix, cooked
1 Tbsp	flaxseed meal
1 Tbsp	grated ginger root
2 Tbsp	org. lemon juice
	chili powder, cilantro, cumin & coriander to taste

Salads & Dressings

8 Gourmet Tropical Salad

1		large banana, sliced
1		mango, 3/8" dice
2 c		pineapple, fresh, 1/2" diced
		juice of 1 guava
2		kiwifruit, sliced 1/8", remove skin
16		Brazil nuts
1/4 c		pumpkin seeds (pepitas)
1/2 c		cashews
16		dates, halved
1/3 lb (1 c)		macadamia nuts
14 oz		Salsa
1 3"		jicama, 3/8" dice
1/2 cup		agave nectar
1 tsp		jalapeno, minced
1/4 cup		apple cider vinegar
1 cup		red bell pepper, 3/8" dice
dash		cayenne pepper

Combine banana, mango, pineapple, guava juice, kiwifruit, and dates, and mix.
Combine salsa ingredients, mix thoroughly.
Top salad with salsa mixture, and garnish with nuts and pepitas.

9 Gratest Salad   7/29/2014

1	avocado, diced
3	carrots, grated
2 inch	beet, grated
1/2 cup	coconut, shredded
1	lime, halved, end stems removed, juiced into salad, then julienned 1/8"
1/8 cup	sunflower seeds, raw
1/2 cup	radish-red clover sprouts
1 large	red bell pepper, sliced into 4 sections, julienned 1/4"
8	crimini mushrooms, 1/8" sliced
1 large	garlic clove, minced
1 cup	romaine lettuce, 1" x 2" strips
4	pear or grape tomatoes, 1/8" sliced
1 large	cucumber, grated
1 1/2 cups	yellow squash, grated (about 1/2 the squash)
2 cups	spinach-&-early spring greens mix
2 Tbsp	ginger root, grated
1 Tbsp	dill seed

Sauce

2 Tbsp	Seeds of Change "Jalfrezi" Curry sauce
4 Tbsp	Bragg Liquid Aminos
1/8 cup(+)	extra virgin olive oil
4 drops	Tabasco sauce

Mix together well & serve cool. Makes about 3/4 gallon.

Salads & Dressings

10 Indian Salad 6.23.2015
1 head	red salad savoy cabbage, julienne
1/2 cup	red onion, 1/2" diced
2 Tbsp	ginger, chopped
1	shallot, sliced
2	leeks, split down middle, sliced 1/8"
1 bunch	cilantro, chopped
1	yellow squash, halved, sliced
1 16 oz jar	Taste of India Hyderabadi Korma Rich Cashew & Cumin cooking sauce
1 can	Thai Kitchen coconut milk, original
1 tsp	cardamom pods
1/4 cup	sunflower seeds
15 oz can	great northern beans
1/4 tsp	parsley, fresh
1/4 tsp	sage, fresh
1/4 tsp	dill, fresh
	salt & pepper to taste

11 Italian Leek Salad
1 c	garbanzo beans, soaked 8 hours (or cooked)
1 c	cannellini beans, soaked 8 hours (or cooked)
1	large leek, 1/4" slices
2	small zucchinis, sliced 1/4" thick
1	4" Portabello mushroom, in 3/4" cubes
1 cup	Italian parsley, chopped
3	garlic cloves, thinly sliced
1	red onion, 3/4" diced
2 Tbsp	fennel seed
5 oz	baby Romaine leaves
12.7 oz	Meditalia Basil Pesto (vegan)
1 Tbsp	Italian seasoning
	olive oil

Directions: Layer romaine on bottom. Top with beans, then zucchini and leeks. Sprinkle mushroom over beans, zucchini and leeks.
Blend parsley, garlic, onion, pesto, fennel, oil and Italian seasoning together, and drizzle over salad.   Makes about 12 cups. (3/4 gallon)

12 Mediterranean Salad
1 head	Romaine lettuce, in roughly 1" squares
1 c	peperoncini, whole, no artificial coloring added
1/2 cup	Kalamata olives, pitted
1/2 cup	pine nuts
1/2 cup	red onion, sliced
1/4 c	basil leaves, fresh, whole
1	garlic clove, chopped
1/2 cup	extra-virgin olive oil (dressing)
1/4 cup	organic balsamic vinegar (dressing) (opt.)
1 cup	artichoke hearts, slightly mashed

Rub bowl with garlic clove, & toss romaine, basil, artichokes, olives, garlic & pine nuts together in the bowl. (Cut off end slice of garlic used to rub bowl). Garnish with peperoncini and onion. Mix olive oil and balsamic vinegar and drizzle over salad.

Salads & Dressings

13 Mint-Apple-Kiwi Salad
4	2.5-3.5 inch apple, 1/4" wedges
4	kiwi fruit, 1/4" slices, cut width-wise
1 cup	blueberries
4	fresh peppermint or spearmint leaves

Arrange in shallow 6" dessert dishes alternating apples and kiwi fruit in one layer. Then place 1/4 c of blueberries in center, and garnish with mint leaf. Serves 4.

14 Mexican Tortilla Casserole--2018
2 12-pack	6 inch yellow corn tortillas
1 15-oz can	black beans
1 15-oz can	pinto beans
1 15-oz can	kidney beans
8 med-large	romaine leaves, julienned
1	red bell pepper, julienned
2	tomatillos, small dice
1+ 16-oz jar	chili verde sauce
1 32-oz jar	enchilada sauce or similar sauce
1/2 cup	red onion, medium dice
1/2 bunch	cilantro, coarsely chopped
2	limes, 1 for juice, cut 1 into 6-8 wedges for garnish (middle and corners)
1	avocado, skinned and 1/4-inch sliced

Directions: Wipe 9x13 casserole dish with olive oil, and pour about 2/3 of enchilada sauce into bottom of casserole dish. Follow with 1/4 of chili verde sauce. Layer tortillas in over-lapping fashion on top of sauce in a 2x3 pattern. Place kidney beans and onions on top of this first layer. Place 2nd layer of tortillas in same fashion, with pinto beans and tomatillos on top of tortillas. Place 3rd layer of tortillas, then place black beans and red bell peppers on top. Top with 4th layer of tortillas and remainder of verde and enchilada sauce. Bake at 200 for 15 minutes. Let cool, and spread romaine and cilantro over top, garnish with avocado and lime wedges, and squirt lime juice over all of it.

15 Mextravaganza 8/19/2013
2	vine-ripened tomatoes, organic
1 small	jalapeno pepper, sliced
1	red bell pepper, julienne, halved
2	tomatillos, diced
2	avocados, diced
1	sweet long pepper, diced
1	red Fresno pepper, diced
1	3 inch diameter jicama, diced
1/2 cup	red onion, 1/4" dice
2 cloves	garlic, minced
1/2 cup	olive oil
8 large	romaine leaves, cut into strips
2	green onions, chopped
5	key limes with rind of one, flesh & juice of 4
1	medium sweet potato, 1/4" dice
30 oz	pinto beans, prepared
2 Tbsp	oregano
16 oz	yellow kernel corn

Salads & Dressings

Mextravaganza cont'd
- 1 cup — cilantro, fresh
- 1 Tbsp — cumin
- 1 Tbsp — coriander
- 1 Tbsp — paprika

Rinse corn in colander over bowl under warm water for 2 minutes. Combine ingredients and serve.

16 Mini-Mexican Salad
- onion
- avocado
- Anaheim pepper
- assorted peppers
- tomatillos
- zucchini
- frozen vegetables
- jicama
- black beans
- chili beans (kidney, pinto, black)
- peppers

17 Oblivion Salad 4/27/2015
- Arugula
- lettuce blend/spring mix
- carrots
- turnip
- black eye peas
- adzuki beans
- pinto beans
- soaked red quinoa
- orange bell pepper
- turmeric root, grated
- ginger root, grated
- flax seed meal
- kale
- Thai Kitchen coconut milk (original)
- tahini
- garlic cloves
- shallot
- fennel seed
- cayenne pepper
- celery seed
- garam masala
- olive oil
- curry powder
- lemon juice
- crimini mushrooms
- pumpkin seeds
- avocado (sliced for garnish)

Salads & Dressings

18 Pedro's Garden
1 15-oz can	pinto beans
1/2 cup	yellow kernel corn
1	red Anaheim pepper, halved & julienned
1	kale leaf, shredded
3 leaves	sage, fresh, shredded or torn
2 leaves	fresh basil, shredded or torn
1	carrot, sliced on bias
1	large garlic clove, sliced & coarsely chopped
3	crimini mushrooms, sliced
2 Tbsp	olive oil
3 sprigs	parsley, coarsely chopped
	Bragg liquid aminos (opt.)

19 Penne Garden Pasta Salad
16 oz	Tinkyada Brown Rice Penne pasta, cooked
25-32 oz jar	organic Garden Vegetable spaghetti sauce
1/2 oz	dried Portabello mushroom, soaked in warm water 30 minutes
5 oz	organic baby spinach leaves
2 tsp	Italian seasoning
1 cup	dry garbanzo beans, cooked
2	carrots, grated
1	red onion, diced
2 Tbsp	extra virgin olive oil
1	garlic clove

Cook and drain pasta, and heat spaghetti sauce to 100-140 degrees. Combine spaghetti sauce, carrots, red onion, garlic and Italian seasoning, place on pasta, and garnish with spinach leaves, garbanzos and mushrooms.

20 Piquant Mustard Potato Salad (made at Sheraton with guidance from Connor) 11.19.2015
all ingredients are given as quantity according to total weight of potatoes
russet potatoes-cooked until firm but soft enough to eat
red bell pepper-1 per 2 lbs of potatoes, finely chopped
celery-1 rib per pound of potatoes
garlic-4 cloves per pound
red onion-1/4 cup minced per pound
prepared mustard - 1 Tbsp per pound
Dijon mustard - 1/2 cup per pound
1/2 tsp salt per pound
white pepper - 1/2 tsp / pound
dill weed - 1 tsp / pound
oregano - 1 tsp / pound
thyme - 1 tsp / pound
sage - 1 tsp / pound

Salads & Dressings

21 Rainbow Vegetable Salad
Makes 1 gallon

1/2 head	Romaine lettuce, 1" strips
1/2 head	red cabbage, 1/4" strips
3	medium carrots, sliced
1/2 cup	red onion, 3/8" dice
1	avocado, sliced
1	medium sweet potato, skin removed, 3/8" dice
2 Tbsp	ginger, fresh, grated
1	red bell pepper, cut in 4ths, julienne strips
9	artichoke hearts, sliced into thirds
3	garlic cloves, minced
1/2 cup	cilantro leaves, fresh, stemmed, coarsely chopped
1	lime, with zest and wedged
3 Tbsp	Dash-o-Dill seasoning
	extra-virgin olive oil

1. Mix romaine, red cabbage, carrots, onions, pepper and artichokes.
2. Boil sweet potato until tender, about 15 minutes.
3. Combine garlic, ginger, dash-o-dill, cilantro and olive oil, whisk and set aside.
4. Dice sweet potato, and sprinkle on salad mixture, add sliced avocado, and lime, then drizzle herb dressing onto potato mixture.

22 Salad with Almonds & Sprouts
radishes
spinach
kale
romaine
red bell pepper
broccoli
carrots
sugar snap peas
artichokes
garbanzo beans
avocado
cucumber
red onion, minced
ginger root
sprouts (legume, mixed)
sliced almonds
Dash-o-dill seasoning(dill weed, garlic, onion, orange peel, sesame seed)

23 Salad for a King

10 leaves	Romaine lettuce
5	white mushrooms, sliced
1 stalk	Broccoli, cut into bite-sized pieces
10 leaves	Red cabbage, shredded
2 leaves	Kale, shredded
3 oz	baby greens (Mesclun, or early spring mix)
1	cucumber, sliced
1	carrot, sliced
2 oz	fresh spinach leaves, julienne
1/2 cup	red onion, chopped

Salads & Dressings

Salad for a King, cont'd
- 1/8 cup — fresh ginger, sliced 1/8 inch (8-10 slices)
- 1/4 cup dry — mung beans, sprouted
- 4 — artichoke hearts
- 1/4 cup dry — black-eyed peas, cooked
- 1/4 cup dry — black beans
- 1/4 cup dry — garbanzo beans
- 2 Tbsp — pesto (dairy-free)
- 10 — Kalamata olives, pitted
- 2 — garlic cloves, thinly sliced
- 1 tsp — curry powder
- 2 Tbsp — fennel seed
- 1 Tbsp — Italian seasoning
- 1 Tbsp — fresh rosemary
- 1 tsp — Dash-o-Dill seasoning, (or 1 tsp fresh or dried dill weed)
- extra virgin olive oil

24 Salad with Pesto & Pizzazz
- 10 leaves — Romaine
- 5 — white mushrooms (button)
- 1 stalk — broccoli
- 10 leaves — red cabbage, shredded
- 2 leaves — Kale
- 2.5 oz — baby greens
- 1 — cucumber
- 1 — carrot
- 2 oz — baby spinach leaves
- 1/3 cup — red onion, sliced
- 1/8 c — fresh ginger root, 1/8" slices
- 1/4 c dry — mung beans, sprouted
- 1/3 c — artichoke hearts
- 1/4 c dry — blackeye peas
- 1/4 c dry — black beans
- 1/4 c dry — garbanzo beans
- 1-3 Tbsp — pesto (see Pickles,Relish,Salsa & Sauce)
- 10 — Kalamata olives, pitted
- 2 cloves — garlic, thinly sliced
- 1 tsp — curry powder
- 2 Tbsp — fennel seed
- 1 Tbsp — Italian seasoning
- 1 Tbsp — rosemary
- 1 tsp — Dash-o-dill seasoning
- 1 — jalapeno, sliced
- 1 — feijoa or guava, thinly sliced
- 1/4 c — arugula lettuce, coarsely chopped
- 1 — red radish "flower" for garnish
- 1/4 tsp — apple cider vinegar spritz
- juice of 1 lime
- 1/2 tsp — aloe vera juice spritz

Salads & Dressings

25   Salad
- Romaine
- carrots
- kale
- zucchini
- cucumbers
- spinach
- sugar snap peas
- red cabbage
- bell peppers
- burdock
- alfalfa
- radish
- red clover
- thyme
- basil
- oregano
- red peppers

26 Spinach Salad 3.15.2015
- spinach
- pecans
- Granny Smith apple, cored, sliced with peel on
- caramelized red onions in brown sugar

27 Summer Fruit Jazz (Salad)

2	strawberries
10	blueberries
1	kiwifruit
1 cup	pineapple, fresh
10	raspberries
1	guava
1	starfruit
1/4 cup	pomegranate
1/4 cup	papaya flesh
1 Tbsp	apple cider vinegar
1 Tbsp each	lemon juice & lime juice

Salads & Dressings

28   Super Salad (salad bar)
      1   alfalfa/bean sprouts
      2   artichokes
      3   avocado or guacamole
      4   beets
      5   bell peppers
      6   broccoli
      7   cabbage (red and/or green)
      8   carrots
      9   celery
    10   cucumbers
    11   garbanzo beans
    12   green onions
    13   jicama/pico de gallo
    14   kidney beans
    15   Mesclun mix (early spring greens)
    16   mushrooms
    17   olives (black and/or green)
    18   peas and/or sugar snap peas
    19   red onions
    20   red radish
    21   Romaine lettuce
    22   snow peas
    23   spinach
    24   water chestnuts
    25   yellow squash
    26   zucchini

29   The Salad Bar
    Romaine lettuce
    garbanzo beans
    kidney beans
    beets
    peas
    carrots
    cucumbers
    zucchini
    yellow squash
    spinach
    cherry or grape tomatoes
    sunflower seeds
    bell peppers (red, orange, yellow, green)
    sprouts
    mushrooms
    (fresh fruit)
    pico de gallo (may substitute for tomatoes)

Salads & Dressings

30 Tropical Tango Fruit Salad (22 fruits)
1. acerola (confirm quantity)
2. carambola (remove black seeds)
3. dragonfruit
4. feijoa
5. goji berry (confirm quantity)
6. guava
7. kiwifruit
8. kumquat
9. lychee
10. mandarin orange
11. mango
12. mangosteen
13. noni
14. papaya
15. pineapple
16. starfruit
17. passionfruit
18. quince
19. Asian pear
20. Tamarillo
21. Kiwano melon
22. pepino

31 Ukrainian beet salad
13 oz	red beets, fresh, diced 1/4"
5 oz	green peas, fresh
10 oz	cabbage, shredded
1-1/2 oz	cucumbers, diced 1/4"
3 oz	onion, diced 1/4"
1 Tbsp	fennel seed
1 oz (1/8 cup)	olive oil

DRESSINGS

1D #1 Honey-Mustard Dressing
1/2 c	olive oil
1/4 c	honey
1/2 tsp	turmeric
1/2 tsp	curry powder
1 tsp	yellow mustard seed powder
1/8 tsp	ginger root
1 wedge	1/6 or 1/8 of a fresh lemon, with rind, zested or finely grated
1/8 tsp	lemon pepper

Combine ingredients, and hand-mix, for "home-made" touch, or whip in blender to emulsify. Delicious!

2D Creamy Fiesta Honey-Mustard Dressing
1/8 c	soymilk or other non-dairy milk beverage
1/8 c	salsa (tomato, jicama, jalapeno, cilantro, red onion)
1-2 Tbsp	honey
1/2 tsp	horseradish root
1/8 c	Dijon mustard (or, yellow mustard, apple cider vinegar, honey)

Salads & Dressings

3D Green Goddess Dressing   (literally!)
1	medium cucumber
4 sprigs	parsley
4	basil leaves, large fresh
2 sprigs	rosemary, fresh
2 oz	alfalfa sprouts
4	peppermint leaves, fresh
4 oz	aloe vera juice
2 sprigs	thyme, fresh
1 sprig	dill weed, fresh
1	celery stalk with leaves
1 stalk	green onions
1 Tbsp	lemon juice
1 Tbsp	raw apple cider vinegar
1/2 c	olive oil

4D Honey Mustard Dressing
1-1/2 cup	olive oil
3/4 cup	water
1/2 cup	apple cider vinegar
5 Tbsp	honey
5 Tbsp	yellow mustard seed powder
2 Tbsp	lemon juice
2 tsp	ginger root
1	garlic clove
1/4 tsp	sea salt
1/4 tsp	turmeric
1/8 tsp	cayenne powder

5D Sweet & Tangy Raspberry Vinaigrette
3/8 cup	Apple Cider Vinegar
3/8 cup	Red wine vinegar
2 cups	raspberries, whole (fresh or frozen)
1-1/2 cups	canola oil (for storage in refrigerator)
2 Tbsp	brown sugar
1/2 cup	honey

Puree first 3 ingredients until creamy. Add canola oil* until mixture is homogenized. Add honey and sugar separately, to taste. A delicate match of sweetness and pungency, without being overpowering. Makes 1 quart.
* or other refrigerator-stable oil

6D Raspberry-Grapeseed Oil Vinaigrette
1 c	raspberries, pureed
1/2 c	apple cider vinegar
1/2 c	organic balsamic vinegar
1 c	Grapeseed oil
1 c	extra-virgin olive oil

Note: This recipe is best for those who appreciate the unique taste of Grapeseed oil and a pungent flavor, since the only sweet is the raspberries, plus the piquant flavor of the . apple cider vinegar.

7D Phil's Famous Yogurt Dressing

    1 qt   plain yogurt
    1 Tbsp onion powder
    1 tsp   garlic powder
    1 tsp   lemon-pepper
    1 Tbsp parsley flakes

Additions: Fiesta Ranch--1/4 tsp each cumin, coriander, chili powder
           honey-mustard--2 Tbsp honey, 3 Tbsp dry mustard

Combine ingredients (yogurt, onion powder, garlic powder, lemon-pepper, parsley flakes.)
Stir or whisk until well-blended and creamy.
Add "extras" if desired. Serve with vegetables, salad, etc.

Smoothies

Basic
1	banana
8 oz	Green Goodness
4 oz	Multi-V
1	kiwifruit
1/4 cup	pumpkin seeds
1/8 cup	almonds
1 Tbsp	lecithin
1/4 tsp	ginger root, slice
1/8 tsp	cinnamon

#2 Superfruit Basic
- banana
- Green Goodness (all 3 juices from Bolthouse Farms)
- Berry Boost or Multi-V
- Acai + 10
- soy lecithin
- kiwi fruit
- almonds
- sunflower seeds
- garam masala
- nutritional yeast

Combine all ingredients in blender. Mix until smooth. Serve in large glass.

#3 Pomegranate-Acai
- banana
- Green Goodness
- Pomegranate & Acai (Lakewood)
- dulse
- almonds
- pecans
- pumpkin seeds
- soy lecithin
- kiwifruit
- blueberries
- raspberries

#4 Digestive Dynamo
- banana
- whole pineapple
- whole papaya
- almonds
- pumpkin seeds
- Berry Boost

#5 Enzyme-Vita-Meister
- papaya
- banana
- mango
- ginger root
- raw sunflower seeds
- Granny Smith apple, (without core)
- fresh parsley
- Acai+10 juice

Smoothies

General ingredients
Fruit
banana
fruit juice (berries and/or yellow-orange fruit)
kiwifruit
raspberries
blueberries
pineapple(whole, yellow flesh)
papaya(whole, flesh w/o seeds)
Acai + 10
Pomegranate & Acai
Blue Machine
C-Boost
Knudsen Morning Blend
Knudsen Lemon Ginger Echinacea
Amazing Mango or equivalent
cranberries
apples
orange
zante currants

Veggies, Nuts, Etc.
Naked Juice Green Machine
Bolthouse Farms Green Goodness (more nutrient-dense than Naked Juice)
almonds
pecans
sunflower seeds
soy lecithin
nutritional yeast
dulse flakes
soy protein powder
soymilk or coconut milk, etc.
molasses(unsulphured)
pumpkin seeds
garam masala
cinnamon
allspice
5-spice powder
turmeric
garlic cloves
(limited to your imagination)
raw ingredients of juices mentioned
medicinal herbs (ginseng, milk thistle powder, etc.)
acerola cherry
rosehips
other dry or liquid nutritional supplements
Garden of Life Protein powder/Raw Meal

Soups & Stews

1 Borscht

1 gallon	vegetable stock(1 gallon water w/3 following ingredients)
2 c	carrots, grated
2 c	celery, sliced
2 c	onion, chopped
6 c	beets, grated
2 c	cabbage, shredded
2 c	spinach, shredded
4	garlic cloves, minced
1/2 c	parsley leaves, fresh
1 c	olive oil
	sea salt & black pepper to taste

In a 6-quart pot, sauté carrots, celery and onion in 1/4 cup olive oil, until onions are golden.
Add water. Prepare cabbage, spinach, beets, and stir in.
Simmer over medium heat for 15-60 minutes to blend flavors. Stir in parsley and garlic
5 minutes before end of cooking time. Remove from heat, and serve.

2 Butternut Squash Stew 6.30.17

1	garlic clove
1	leek
2	carrots
1	celery stalk
	olive oil
	(Saute above ingredients)
1	butternut squash, peeled & cubed (or frozen cubed butternut squash)
1	anise/fennel stalk w/stems & fronds
6 oz jar	marinated artichokes
2 Tbsp	fresh basil
1	zucchini
1	red bell pepper
7 cups	cold water
2	collard leaves
2 cups	red cabbage
1 15-oz can	pinto beans
1 15-oz can	cannellini beans
12	tarragon leaves
8	sage leaves
2 Tbsp	dry rosemary
2 Tbsp	fenugreek powder
	red, white & black quinoa blend

3 Cold Annihilating Soup

1 qt	purified water
2 Tbsp	garlic, granulated, or 2 garlic cloves, sliced
2 Tbsp	cayenne pepper
1 pkg.	vegetable broth or soup
20 leaves	parsley, fresh
2	peppermint leaves, fresh
1 tsp	black pepper

Bring water to boil; add all ingredients and reduce heat to medium-high. After 5 minutes,
reduce heat, and simmer for 5 minutes or longer, depending on your "spice
threshold".

Soups & Stews

4 Corn Chowder   need 8-12 quart pan or stock pot.
- 1 gallon   vegetable stock (1 cup each carrots, celery, onions) with sufficient water
- 32 oz   sweet yellow kernel corn
- 2 lbs   Russet, Red, and/or Yukon Gold potatoes, 3/8" diced
- 2 c   carrots, sliced
- 1/2 c   almond milk
- 1   red bell pepper, diced 1/4"
- 2 c   celery, sliced
- 1/2 c   white onion, chopped
- 1 c   olive oil
- 1/2 tsp   sea salt
- 1/4 c   garbanzo bean flour (thickener)

Sauté onions, celery and carrots until onions are transparent. Add potatoes, carrots, celery and onions, and 1 gallon water. Cook until potatoes are just starting to get soft, about 30 minutes, on medium heat. Add corn, almond milk and red pepper. Cook for 10-15 minutes, add salt and garbanzo flour. Cook for another 5-10 minutes until flour is absorbed, and soup is desired thickness. Serve.

5 Creole Southern Gumbo 10.14.17
- 8 inch   sweet potato, cubed
- 1 cup   long grain brown rice, dry
- 1/2 cup   black-eye peas, dry
              (cook brown rice and black eye peas 15 minutes first)
- 1/8 tsp   cayenne
- 1 tsp   allspice
- 1 Tbsp   Gumbo file seasoning (sassafras & thyme)
- 4 tsp   garlic cloves
- 1 cup   red onion, diced
- 1/4 cup   white onion, diced
- 1   green bell pepper, diced
- 1   red bell pepper, diced
- 1 cup   raw okra, sauteed 3-6 minutes in olive oil, placed into mix in final 15 minutes)
- 15 oz can   red beans
- 15 oz can   black beans
- 3 cups   collards, 1/2 inch strips, steamed 1 minute
- 2 Tbsp   ginger root, grated
- 2 cups   cold water

6 German Cabbage & Apples (Four Points by Sheraton, Kiwanis Christmas Party) 12.15.2015
for 24 people
- 8   apples, 1/8 inch sliced
- 8 pounds   red cabbage, shredded
- 8 Tbsp   brown sugar
- 2-2/3 cup   red wine vinegar
- 8 tsp   salt
- 8 Tbsp   bacon fat (from 36 strips of cooked bacon) or thick aromatic oil for sautéing
- 1/2 cup   minced onions
- 4   onions, peeled & pierced with 2 cloves per onion
- 4   bay leaves
- 4 cups   boiling water

Soups & Stews

German Cabbage & Apples, cont'd
Put cabbage in large bowl, add vinegar, salt & sugar. Toss until coated. Melt bacon fat or oil in pot, cook minced onions and apples 5 minutes.
Add cabbage, whole onions and bay leaves. Bring the 4 cups of water to boil, add to cabbage mixture, and bring mixture to a boil, stirring occasionally.
Reduce heat to Low and simmer 1 hour. Remove onions and bay leaves before serving.

7   Hearty Cold-Day Soup 1.2018
        quinoa
        old-world pilaf
        millet
        carrot
        young kale
        rosemary
        GF dumplings (GF flour & water)
        red & white onion, diced
        red or yellow potato
        1-2 ribs celery
        3-4 garlic cloves
        oregano
        Italian seasoning
        olive oil

8   Gumbo   9.28.2013

1 gallon	cool water
1/2 cup	long grain brown rice
1/2 cup	black beans
2	Roma tomatoes, 1/4" diced
1 stalk	celery, 1/8" sliced
1 cup	fresh okra, 1/2" sliced
1/4 cup	sorghum flour (roux)
2	garlic cloves, minced
1 Tbsp	olive oil
1	red bell pepper, 1/4" diced
1/4 cup	red onion, minced
3	bay leaves (remove before serving)--put leaves in teaball, place in soup
1 Tbsp	fennel seed
dash	cayenne pepper
1 tsp	oregano
1 Tbsp	sage
1/8 tsp	coriander
1/8 tsp	equal mix of black pepper, bell peppers, mustard seed, sea salt
1 Tbsp	fresh ginger root, finely grated
2 Tbsp	gumbo file powder
dash	sea salt

Soups & Stews

> **Directions** NOTE: Add okra LAST, to prevent the soup from getting "gooey" from the mucilaginous qualities of the okra. Make sure beans are fully cooked, if dry. Baking recommended.
>
> **Directions** Sauté the "mirepoix" (oil, garlic, onion, carrot and celery), then your herbs and spices, for about 10 minutes, then gradually stir in vegetables, rice, "roux", file powder, then in the last 10-15 minutes, add the okra, after rice is cooked. Cook another 5 minutes on low heat, remove from heat, and serve.
>
> NOTE: If using meat, brown it while sautéing the stock. Cook only until light brown (as in the case of Andouille sausage), as it will have a chance to cook for another 20-30 minutes and help flavor the soup.

9 Hash with Cubed Beef (my version, Sheraton Hotel, BBQ Night, 8.20.2014)

16 lbs	beef	(or Shiitake or Portabello mushrooms, legumes, nuts, at appropriate weight)
10	Russet potatoes, 3/8" dice	
3	yellow onions: 3/8" dice	
3 red, 2 green	bell peppers, chopped	
5 cloves	garlic, minced	
4 stalks	celery, minced	
4 Tbsp	horseradish (prepared with vinegar only)	
1 Tbsp	dry yellow mustard	
3 Tbsp	thyme	
1 Tbsp	celery salt	
2 Tbsp	black pepper	
1 Tbsp	Kosher or sea salt	

Note: This recipe may need some working over for "proper texture".

Directions: Wash & cut vegetables. Prepare a large brazing pan or skillet with olive oil, turned to medium-high heat. (If using legumes, make sure to presoak or pre-cook them to suitable level of softness before cooking with remainder of vegetables.)

Place potatoes in pan, and cook for 20 minutes until soft. Add remainder of vegetables, and herbs and spices, and cook until potatoes are al dente and ready to eat, with a golden brown color.

10 Melon Soup

4 c	watermelon, 3/4" balled
4 c	honeydew or musk melon, 3/4" balled
4 c	casaba, 3/4" balled
4 c	cantaloupe, 3/4" balled
4 c	crenshaw, 3/4" balled
2 c	honeydew, pureed
2 c	aloe vera juice
	peppermint sprigs to garnish

Peel melons with knife, remove seeds with spoon. Use melon-baller to scoop out 3/4" balls until no more melon is left. Scoop out and puree remaining melon flesh.

Soups & Stews

11 Mexican Minestrone
Add to 1 gallon cool water in 6-quart pan:
- 2 celery ribs, halved and sliced
- 1/4 cup white onion, chopped
- 1/4 cup red onion, chopped
- 16 oz sweet kernel corn, frozen
- 2 yellow squash, sliced
- 1/4 cup red quinoa, uncooked
- 1 red Fresno pepper, chopped
- 1 jalapeno, minced
- 1 orange bell pepper, diced
- 2 Tbsp cumin
- 1 tsp coriander
- 2 Tbsp oregano
- 1-3 tsp Stonemill Essentials Chicken & Poultry Grinder (black peppercorns, mustard seed, onion, salt, garlic, green and red bell pepper (to taste)
- 1 tsp garlic, minced
- dash chili powder
- dash cayenne pepper
- 2 Roma tomatoes
- 16 oz black beans, or 1 15-oz can
- 1 cup garbanzo beans, dry, or 15 oz can
- 1/2 cup fresh cilantro, loose
- 1 avocado, mashed
- 1/2 cup Bob's Red Mill Garbanzo-Fava flour (thickener)

1 Sauté onions & celery, add corn, squash, peppers, dry seasonings. Simmer over medium heat for 20 minutes until squash is tender. Stir in quinoa, garlic & beans. Simmer for 10 minutes. Add tomatoes and Gar-fava flour, stir & simmer for another 10 minutes. Remove from heat. Stir in cilantro, & top with avocado.

12 Minestrone -Sweet Potato Savoy
- 3 stalks celery, sliced
- 3 garlic cloves, large, sliced
- 2 Tbsp olive oil
- 2 Russet potatoes, 1/2" dice
- 1 zucchini, 1/2" dice
- 2 qts water
- 2 carrots, sliced
- 32 oz garbanzo beans or cannellini beans
- 2 Tbsp rosemary, dried
- 1 Tbsp Tabasco sauce (opt.)
- 1 Tbsp basil, dried
- 1 sweet potato, 1/2" dice
- 1 c savoy cabbage
- 1/2 cup white onion, 1/4" dice

Directions: Bring water to medium heat, adding carrots, onions, celery and oil. Allow to simmer for 5-10 minutes. Add cabbage, zucchini, beans and herbs, stir, and allow to simmer for about 30 minutes to 1 hour or longer. 10 minutes before serving, stir in garlic, and let simmer for remaining time. Makes about 1-1/2 gallons of soup.

Soups & Stews

13 Minestrone-Butternut Squash & Mushroom
2/3 cup	garbanzo beans
2/3 cup	cannellini beans
2	carrots, diced
1	turnip, diced
½ head	red cabbage, shredded into ½ inch x 2 inch strips
1	Portabello, or 3 button, crimini or porcini mushrooms, ½ inch dice
¼ cup	fresh curly or Italian parsley
1	Butternut squash, ½ inch dice HINT: cut in half and slice off skin-rind with knife
3	garlic cloves, thinly sliced
1 Tbsp	Italian seasoning
1 tsp	fennel seed

Put 1 gallon of water into 6-quart pot, set to medium heat, add carrots, garlic and fennel seed. Let simmer while cutting vegetables. Put butternut squash into pot, then Portabello mushrooms, turnips and cabbage, followed by Italian seasoning. Stir, and add beans and parsley. Reduce heat to medium-low, let simmer up to 30-60 minutes. Serve hot.

14 Potato Soup
2	Russet potatoes, large, skin-on, 3/4" diced
6	Russet potatoes, large, skin-on, pureed
2	Yukon Gold potatoes, skin-on, 1/2" diced
5	Yukon Gold potatoes, skin-on, pureed
2	Red potatoes, skin-on, 1/2" diced
4	Red potatoes, skin-on, pureed
2	Red bell peppers, diced
2	celery ribs with leaves, chopped
2	carrots, sliced
1	white onion, diced
2	garlic cloves, chopped
2 Tbsp	paprika
2 Tbsp	parsley, fresh, coarsely chopped
1 Tbsp	dill weed
2 Tbsp	green onions, sliced 1/4"

Soups & Stews

15 Spicy Vegetarian Chili

16 oz each	kidney, black & pinto beans, dry
16 oz	garbanzo beans
16 oz	anasazi beans (opt.)
1	large tomato, chopped
3	jalapeno peppers, diced 1/4"
2	carrots, grated
1/2 cup	molasses
8 oz	yellow corn kernels
1 Tbsp	cayenne powder
1	red onion, diced 1/2"
1 Tbsp	cumin (may use seed)
1/8 c	cilantro, coarsely chopped
1 Tbsp	coriander
1 Tbsp	black pepper
4	garlic cloves, sliced
4 oz	habanero pepper salsa, or 1 habanero pepper, grated
2 Tbsp	oregano
1	red bell pepper, diced 1/2"

Put beans, seasoning and pepper sauce into 6-quart pan, turn on to low heat. Prepare vegetables, dice jalapenos, red bell pepper, red onion, chop cilantro. Place remaining ingredients into pot and let cook for 4-6 hours. Serves 8.

16 Vegetable-Bean Stew 11.11.17

saute 2 cloves garlic, 1 carrot & 1/4 c red onion in olive oil

1	zucchini, halved & sliced
	Add 2 cups cool water
1	orange bell pepper
3	small beets
1 Tbsp	Italian seasoning
1/2 tsp	dried rosemary
1 Tbsp	parsley
1 Tbsp	cilantro
1 medium	potato, diced (Russet, Yukon Gold, Red, Blue,…)
2 Tbsp	cumin
1 tsp	turmeric
1 tsp	Worcestershire sauce
2 tsp	Dijon mustard
1 cup	wild rice blend
1 cup	Italian green beans
1/2 cup	red lentils
1/2 cup	buckwheat groats
1 tsp	dry minced garlic
30 oz	pinto beans, cooked/prepared
1/4 cup	flaxseed meal
1 tsp	gumbo file (thyme & sassafras)
	salt & pepper to taste
dash	cayenne

Soups & Stews

17 Vegetable Potato Soup   11.21.13

Add to 1 gallon cool water:

4	Yukon Gold potatoes, 3/4" dice
2	large carrots
1/4 cup	red onion, chopped
1/2 cup	garbanzo beans, dry
1 Tbsp	fenugreek seed
2 Tbsp	parsley flakes
1	celery rib, 1/8" sliced
1/8 cup	Old World Pilaf
1/8 cup	millet
1/8 tsp	saffron
1 tsp	curry powder, salt-free
1/2 tsp	lemon-ginger tea, dry
2 cloves	garlic, chopped
1 Tbsp	Italian seasoning
1/2 cup	Italian green beans
1 leaf	fresh sage, cut into 1/4" pieces
2 sprigs	fresh thyme
1/3 cup	yellow kernel corn

Add dry herbs, onion and garlic with olive oil to stockpot, saute until onions are almost translucent. Add water, then vegetables and fenugreek seed, and stir. Reduce heat to medium to medium-low, and allow to steep for at least 30 minutes to an hour. Add fresh herbs, let steep another 5-10 minutes. Remove from heat and serve hot.

other ideas: Flaming Texan Chili   Hearty Wild Rice Soup

Vegetables

1 Chef-School Vegetable Stir-Fry

1 c	snow peas
1 c	carrots, sliced
1 c	celery, sliced
1 c	broccoli florets, chopped into bite-size pieces
1 c	bamboo shoots
1/8 c	ginger root, grated or sliced
1 c	cashews, raw or roasted
1 c	green onions, chopped
8 oz	firm tofu, diced 1/2" (8 oz = 1 cup), or 1 package
1 c	onions, diced or sliced
1 c	Purple Emperor's Forbidden Rice (opt.)
1 c	brown basmati rice, or long grain brown jasmine rice
1 c	soy sauce (Bragg's Liquid Aminos)
1/2 c	sesame oil (refined, for frying)

Cook rice for 30 minutes in a 1:3 rice-water ratio over medium-high heat. Combine remaining ingredients except tofu into large skillet. Sauté in oil over medium heat for 10-20 minutes until vegetables are soft but still a bit crisp. Add tofu to vegetable mix, cook for about 5 minutes until tofu absorbs flavors. Top the rice with vegetable mix and serve. Makes 11 cups.

2 Creole Dinner 7.6.2015

2 oz	pimentos
3 cloves	garlic
1	red bell pepper
1	green bell pepper
1	white onion/Vidalia
1/4 cup	grated ginger root
1	sweet potato
1 bunch	collard greens
1 lb.	long grain brown rice
30 oz	black beans, prepared
1	avocado
1/8 tsp	cayenne
4	chives, fresh, chopped
	cumin to taste
	allspice to taste
	parsley to taste
1/8 tsp	salt
1/2 tsp	black pepper

Vegetables

3 East-Indian Shepherd's Pie

10 oz	"JYOTI" classic masala curry sauce or equivalent (or make from scratch)
2	carrots, sliced
1	zucchini, sliced thin
1	red bell pepper, julienne half-length 1/4"
1	celery stalk, sliced
2	garlic cloves, sliced
16 oz	garbanzo beans/chick peas
1	tomato, chopped
1/2 tsp	curry powder
1/2 tsp	celery seed
1 tsp	parsley flakes
1/4 c	cardamom pods (open pod and empty contents, discard pods)
1/8 c	olive oil
1/2 c	garbanzo bean flour (thickening)

Crust:

4 c	garbanzo bean flour
2 c	rice or almond milk
dash	cream of tartar
1 c	olive oil
1/8 tsp	curry powder

1. Prepare vegetables, cook garbanzo beans for 30 minutes on medium-high heat. Combine vegetables, herbs and spices with curry sauce, simmer over medium-low heat, stirring occasionally.
2. Combine garbanzo bean flour, milk, cream of tartar, oil and curry powder, and stir together until thick. Oil the inside of a 9x13 casserole dish, and pour of the flour mixture into the bottom of the dish.
3. Combine chickpeas with vegetable/curry mix, and spoon mixture onto crust, then pour the remaining flour mixture on top of the vegetable/curry mix.
4. Bake in 300 degree oven for 15-30 minutes, until top crust is golden.

4 Endive & Lentils with Sunchoke Sauce

1 cup	millet
1 1/2 cups	French green lentils
1	leek, 1/2" slices
2 Tbsp	Fines Herbes
1/8 cup	sunchoke, grated
1 head	Belgian endive, 1" x 1/2" slices
1	red bell pepper, 1/4" x 1" slices
1	zucchini
2	carrots, quartered, 1/4" dice
1/8 cup	sesame seed

Sauce

1/8 cup	sunchoke, grated
1 Tbsp	sesame seed
1/2 cup	almonds and/or walnuts, soaked & creamed
1	Roma tomato, 1/4" dice
3 Tbsp	parsley
1 Tbsp	ginger root, grated
	olive oil

Vegetables

Endive & Lentils with Sunchoke Sauce, cont'd

Directions: Soak lentils and millet in cool water for 7 hours. Remove 3 cups of mixture and cook remainder of mixture until al dente. (1/2 of mixture "sprouted", 1/2 of mixture cooked)

Sauce: Grate ginger and sunchoke, mince, and combine in blender with almonds and walnuts. Slowly add 1 1/8 cup of water while blending, then add sesame seed and parsley, blend until thoroughly mixed and smooth. Add olive oil to all 3 mixtures, and stir in.
Add a bit of lemon juice to millet/lentils to keep fresh, and combine mixtures, mix well. Makes about 1 gallon.

5 Mexican Mojo Salad (medium-heat)   6.16.2015

15-oz can	pinto beans
15-oz can	chili beans (pinto, kidney, black)
15-oz can	garbanzo beans
1 head	romaine lettuce or green leaf lettuce, 1/2" strips
3	carrots, sliced
10 oz	yellow corn kernels
1	red bell pepper, cut in 3rds and julienned
1	red Fresno pepper, halved and sliced
1	jalapeno pepper, halved and chopped
1	Habanero pepper, halved and minced
1	tomatillo, diced
1	zucchini, halved and sliced
1	red onion, diced (1/2" - 3/4")
1/3 cup	flaxseed meal
8-10 oz	Herdez Chili Verde sauce
1 tsp	cumin
1/2 tsp	coriander
	olive oil to taste

Combine all ingredients in a large bowl.

6 Potato Curry (curried fried potatoes)

1	potato (yellow, red, Russet, etc.)
1/8 cup	sesame oil per potato (or to taste)
3 tsp	curry powder (salt-free)
2	garlic cloves, minced
1 Tbsp	Bragg Liquid Aminos

Slice or grate potato(s), stir in sesame oil, garlic, and liquid aminos. Sauté in skillet on medium heat for 5-10 minutes or until potatoes are golden brown.
Makes 1 serving

7 Potato Pancakes   2.23.2013

2 large	Yukon Gold potatoes, shredded (may also combine Yukons with red potatoes)
1 large	sweet potato, shredded
1/8 cup	parsley, dried
	olive oil

Wash & shred(grate) potatoes, mix together in bowl with parsley & oil.
Place mixture into skillet or fry pan over medium heat, turn over when bottom is golden brown.

Vegetables

8 Quinoa-Beet Curry   12.19.2017

1 cup	red quinoa
1/8 cup	amaranth seed
1 cup	green lentils
1	avocado
1	habanero, sliced & chopped
7	button mushrooms
2	beets, sliced
7	beet greens, julienned
2	small carrots
1	red bell pepper
4	garlic cloves
1/2 cup	red onion
	50/50 lettuce blend (spinach, kale & chard)
	To Taste:
	chili powder
	lemon juice
	basil
	ginger
	cumin
	olive oil
	flaxseed meal

9 Spinach Vindaloo Curry   4.14.2015

10 oz	Red Stem spinach
8 oz	sprouted lentil trio(brown, green, red), soaked 15 minutes in water, drained
25 oz	prepared chick peas
13.6 oz can	Thai Kitchen organic. coconut milk
1	red bell pepper, julienne, cut in 3rds
3	carrots, bias-sliced
1/2 cup	chopped red onion
12 oz jar	Spicy Nothings Spicy Tangy Curry Sauce (Vindaloo)
2 Tbsp	fennel seed
1	organic lime and juice, 1/4 tsp grated rind
1 Tbsp	garam masala
2 Tbsp	fenugreek powder
2 Tbsp	turmeric root, grated
2 Tbsp	ginger root, grated
Directions:	Combine spinach, chick peas, pepper, fennel seed, onion and carrots in a large bowl. Add lentils when done soaking.
	Mix together coconut milk, turmeric, ginger, curry sauce, garam masala & fenugreek powder.
	Add lime juice and zest, and mix into salad.
	Makes 1 gallon of salad

Vegetables

10 Sweet Potato with Quinoa Pasta

9	Romaine leaves
9	broccoli florets
8 oz	quinoa veggie pasta, dry
12	Swiss Chard leaves, de-stemmed
1	sweet potato, grated
1/2 cup	zucchini, 3/8" dice
6	Brazil nuts
3 Tbsp	sunflower seeds, raw
1/8 cup	olive oil

Directions: Bring 1 quart of water to boil, add pasta and oil, return to boil, reduce heat to medium. Cook quinoa pasta for 6-8 minutes. Prepare vegetables, and cut leaves into 1/2" strips. Steam Swiss Chard over medium heat for 15 minutes. Drain, rinse with cool water. Drain pasta and rinse with cool water. Combine pasta, greens and zucchini into a bowl, toss until mixed, and for serving 3 people, place 1/3 of mix, and 3 broccoli flowerets onto each plate, then garnish with 1 Tbsp sunflower seeds, and 2 Brazil nuts each.

11 Sweet Potatoes with Wild Rice   1994~

2	sweet potatoes, whole
2	medium carrots, grated
1 cup	wild rice
1 cup	marinara sauce
2-4 leaves	Romaine lettuce or Kale
1 tsp	oregano
1 tsp	rosemary
1 tsp	parsley

1. Scrub and rinse sweet potatoes, slightly cut into top about 1/4 inch. Poke with fork all over, and boil in 3 quarts water for 15-25 minutes, or until a fork can penetrate easily.
2. Cook wild rice in 3 cups water over medium-high heat for 30-40 minutes until slightly chewy but not tough.
3. Warm marinara in pan, and stir in oregano, rosemary and parsley. Grate carrots, and prepare kale or lettuce (need whole leaves).
4. Stir carrots into marinara sauce, slice sweet potatoes in half and divide the wild rice between the two potatoes, in between the two halves, and ladle the marinara onto the wild rice.   Makes a very healthy, satisfying meal. Add walnuts, pecans or other nuts if desired.

Vegetables

12 Sweet Curry Masala Vegetable Stir-fry   6.6.2015
1	Portabella mushroom, halved, cut in 1/4"-3/8" slices
3	medium carrots, bias-cut
3	zucchini, bias-cut
3	red bell peppers, 3/8" julienne
1	red onion, halved, cut in "X"
4 Tbsp	minced garlic (sauté first with oil)
1/3 cup	olive oil
sprigs	fresh rosemary (garnish)
5	red radish "roses" (garnish)

Sauce
2-15 oz cans	cream of coconut
1/2 tsp	red pepper flakes
2 Tbsp	curry powder
1/2 tsp	yellow mustard seed powder
1 tsp	ginger powder
1 Tbsp	fennel seed
2 tsp	garam masala
1 tsp	lemon juice

1. Stir together sauce ingredients in a small (1 quart) bowl. Sauté garlic in olive oil over medium-high heat until golden brown. Add vegetables into large bowl and mix.
2. Add sauce to vegetables and mix until vegetables are thoroughly coated.
3. Pour vegetable-sauce mixture into pan with garlic and oil, cook until carrots are al dente. Makes about 5 plates. Delicious! Sauce has honey-like sweetness and smooth texture.
4. Garnish: tuck sprig of rosemary into fold of radish rose, and place on edge of plate, next to mixture.

May also be served with [brown] basmati rice.

13 Veggie Stir-fry Meals (for KSU Day Lily Club--Sheraton, 7.11.2015)
1	carrots, sliced
1	broccoli, bite-size
1	red & green bell peppers, julienne
2	mushrooms, sliced
1/8 cup	minced garlic

Combine above prepped vegetables, set aside until ready to saute with sauce for service.

Sauce: Mustard seed-basil
2 15-oz cans	Coco Lopez (or equivalent) cream of coconut
3 Tbsp	cilantro
1 Tbsp	curry
2 Tbsp	ginger
1 tsp	celery seed
2 Tbsp	basil
2 Tbsp	fennel seed
1 tsp	brown mustard seed
1/8 cup	sesame seed
2 Tbsp	lemon juice
2 Tbsp	minced garlic

Saute all of above except cream of coconut & sesame seed over medium heat for 10 minutes with enough olive oil to cover bottom of pan. Stir together coconut & sesame seed & set aside. Remove mixture from heat & put into ice bath, stirring for a few minutes.
Combine saute mixture and coconut cream mixture. Mix into vegetables before sautéing.

Recipes for Reformulation

"parmesan"	pine nuts
apple sauce	
beans	stock pot over night w/kombu (seaweed)
Brownies	
cheddar	almonds, pinenuts, paprika; Rendang Curry Sauce, (sauce)
cheesecake	
coleslaw	Vitamix: cabbage, carrots, red cabbage, celery seed, almond milk,
Coleslaw Dressing	Vitamix
creamy dressings	lecithin?
Key Lime pie	almost, July 2013, too much rind/zest
Lemon Bars	millet flour, lemon juice,
Lemon Cream Pie	
Pie Crust	nuts, dates, coconut oil. Did for pecan pie 3/2014. Good, no baking
pies in general	crust and filling
Ranch Dressing	
scones	GF flour, vegan butter (Earth Balance)
sharp cheddar	garlic, almonds, pine nuts, paprika, lemon juice, cayenne
sweet relish (cucumber)	(no alum) ACV, pickling herbs/spices, sea salt,
whipped topping	nut milk or coconut milk

Almond Biscotti

1 c	almonds
1/4 c	dark, bittersweet chocolate/cacao
1/4 c	carob powder
2 Tbsp	honey
2 Tbsp	almond oil (culinary use)
	(check culinary book for directions)

Fennel Biscotti

1/3 c	almonds
1/3 c	hazelnuts
1/3 c	pine nuts
2 Tbsp	fennel seed
1 Tbsp	packed fennel fronds and stalks
1/4 c	honey
	(check culinary book for directions)

Various Miscellaneous Diets

Paleolithic: Original or Caveman diet, Garden of Eden diet (no domesticated animals)
- grain-free
- bean-free
- potato-free
- dairy-free
- sugar-free
- You CAN eat: meat, fish, fruit, veggies, nuts, berries, nut-milks

Solanine Diet: for those with solanine allergies, can include "Bella donna" family
- tomato-free
- potato-free
- bell/chili pepper-free (includes paprika, pimentos, etc.)
- eggplants
- You CAN eat: all other foods
- Reason: chemical in potatoes and tomatoes which cause green color (unripe/sprouting)

Salicylic Acid Diet: allergic to nuts and/or berries
- berry-free
- nut-free
- You CAN eat: all other foods
- Reason: Salicylic Acid, an acid common to tree nuts, bramble berries(i.e. raspberries), strawberries, etc.

Vegetarian:
- meat-free (no chicken, beef, pork, fish or seafood, etc.)
- You CAN eat: all other foods
    - legumes
    - nuts
    - fruits
    - vegetables
    - grains
    - dairy (milk, eggs, cheese)
    - etc.

Vegan:
- meat-free (no chicken, beef, pork, fish or seafood, etc.)
- dairy-free (animal milk, cheese, butter, eggs)
- bee products (animal, technically)
- You CAN eat: all other foods
    - legumes
    - nuts
    - fruits
    - vegetables
    - grains
    - dairy (milk, eggs, cheese)
    - etc.

Recipe Costing~Salads, Dressings

						total svg	total svg	total svg	
Asian Salad	Full Batch(~1 gallon)---retail $ October 2014	Unit	Qty	$/lb	$/oz	$/8-oz	$/16-oz	$/24-oz	
1 head	Napa Cabbage, 1/2 inch strips (yield ~75 leaves)	ea.	75	2.25	0.14	0.66	1.32	1.98	
1	large carrot, match stick cut, about 1-1/2" x 1/8"	ea.	10	1	0.06	0.04	0.08	0.12	
2 oz	ginger root, finely grated	lb	2	9	0.56	0.07	0.14	0.21	
1/2 cup	cilantro, fresh, lightly chopped	sprig	1	18	1.13	0.07	0.14	0.21	
1	large red bell pepper, halved, 1/4 inch julienne	ea.	1	2	0.13	0.01	0.02	0.02	
8 oz	Mung bean sprouts (bulk mung beans)	oz	8	2.79	0.17	0.09	0.17	0.26	
2 oz	brown sesame seed	oz	2	4.39	0.27	0.03	0.07	0.10	
1 cup dry	garbanzo beans, adzuki or soy beans	oz	8	2.5	0.16	0.08	0.16	0.23	
8 oz	Bragg's Liquid Aminos pure soy sauce	oz	8	4.94	0.31	0.15	0.31	0.46	
2 stalks	lemon grass, sliced, 1/2 inch of each end cut off	oz	2	17.4	1.09	0.14	0.27	0.41	
6 oz	shiitake (10 oz frozen, 1/2 oz dry, 6 oz fresh)	oz	6	6.38	0.40	0.15	0.30	0.45	
4 oz	red onion, diced 1/4 inch	oz	4	1.5	0.09	0.02	0.05	0.07	
6 oz	sesame oil, to taste	oz	6	8	0.50	0.19	0.38	0.56	
2 oz	5-spice powder	oz	2	17.9	1.12	0.14	0.28	0.42	
	Total $					1.70	3.39	5.51	
	Cost of goods sold (1 gal. full batch price)					27.16	27.16	27.56	
	Mark-up					295%	295%	272%	
	Potential Menu Price 1					$ 5.00	$ 10.00	15.00	
	potential Menu Price 2					$ 3.00	$ 6.00	$ 9.00	
	mark-up 2					177%	177%	163%	
						8-oz svg	unit translation		
	AP =					0.2	2.00	leaves	
	As-					0.2	2.00	of carrot	
	purchased	AP $				0.75	3/4 tsp		
	1 head cabbage	$ 4.00				1.875	1.8 sprigs		
	12 9" carrots, 2 lb bag	$ 2.00				1.76625	1.75 inches		
	3/4"x3" rhizome ginger	$ 1.50				1/2 oz sprouts	8 individual sprouts?		
	~30 sprigs cilantro	$ 2.25				0.125	3 1/8 tsp		
	~4" x 3" pepper	$ 3.00				1/2 oz (dry)	1/8 cup cooked/soft		
	1/4"x1/8" each mung beans	$ 1.36				1/2 oz	1 Tbsp		
	1/16" individual sesame seeds	$ 0.54				2.25	2 1/4" lemon grass		
	~1/4" each, garbanzo, adzuki or soy beans	$ 1.50	1 Tbsp	1/2 oz		0.375	3/8 oz mushrooms		
	1 16 oz bottle Bragg's Liquid Aminos	$ 4.94	1 tsp	1/6 oz		1.324688	1-1/4" cube of red onion		
	2 18" stalks lemongrass	$ 2.25				0.375	3/4 Tbsp		
	frzn, dry or fresh shiitake mushrooms	$ 6.00				0.125	1/4 Tbsp (1/2 of 1/2 Tbsp)		
	3" dia. onion	$ 1.70							
	1 16 oz bottle sesame oil	$ 8.00							
	bulk powder or in jar (depending on retailer)	$ 2.24							
		$ 41.28							

Bibliography & Suggested Reads

1. Reader's Digest Assoc., Inc. The Complete Illustrated Book of Herbs. New York: Adult Trade Publishing.
2. Encyclopedia Brittanica 2006 CD
3. Encyclopedia of Herbs, Spices & Flavorings
4. Hagman, Bette (1999). The Gluten-Free Gourmet Bakes Bread. New York: Henry Holt & Company
5. Culinary Institute of America (1996). The New Professional Chef, 6th Ed. Wiley & Sons
6. Smolin, L. & Grosvenor, M. (2004) Nutrition: Science & Applications, 3rd Ed. Wiley & Sons; [Esha Food Nutrition Tables]
7. Balch, J. & P. (1997). Prescription for Nutritional Healing, 2nd Ed. New York: Avery/Penguin Putnam
8. Sunset Publishing (1995). Western Garden Book. California
9. Ohnstad, Dianne. Whole Foods Companion.

Commentary Appendix

This section is information that I have heard, read or discovered for myself through experience, work, eating, testing, and various forms of education.

These may have some "punch" due to the author's personality and his convictions on particular issues.

Most of it is advice, some is factual or statistical, and some is a bit of opinion. However, reading these sections may enlighten your knowledge on the subject of health and wellness, especially where it concerns food.

Hopefully, this information, as well as the recipes in the first half of the book will somehow convince you that this lifestyle (animal-free, whole-foods) will produce significantly better health and well-being, **and** lower your medical costs. According to a recent radio ad, more bankruptcies occur due to medical costs than any other factor, including divorce, and foreclosure. That means, we as a nation need to reestablish our lifestyle priorities, and start treating our bodies with more respect. After all, it's the **only** body we have in this lifetime! It comes down to 2 choices:

      1-eat anything now, pay for it later
      2-exercise some discipline with your diet, and watch
      your medical bills (doctor and hospital) go down.
      (also known as "paying it forward")

They say, if a habit is going to stick, you've got to be motivated! Bear in mind that our society is so in-grained (pun intended) in the fiberless food fiasco that it can be difficult sometimes to "re-engineer" certain recipes for healthier outcomes. Having a natural foods store in your town can be a tremendous benefit for those seeking healthy alternatives to the "SAD" diet. The primary, unfortunate, difference between the "SAD" diet and a whole-foods diet is that the SAD diet is cheaper, AT FIRST, but then, it kicks you in the butt [sic], and you're in the doctor's office before you know it. Then you spend on the doctor what you COULD be spending on wholesome delicious food at the grocery store, and spending too much money on medical insurance because you don't know how to properly take care of your body. Then again, a good grocery store (or farmer's market) with a large fruit and vegetable section, as well as nuts and seeds, will slim you down, **and** give you more energy!

I know it's hard to teach an old dog new tricks sometimes, but I have tried to make at least MOST of the recipes in this book appetizing, to replace the low-energy "comfort" food that the media and deep-pocket food factories sell us, and that often our family and friends try to convince us to eat. "Popular" doesn't mean it's good.

Time to laugh: There's a food joke that goes something like this:
There are some people who will never need to be embalmed after they die, because what they've been eating all along is so full of sodium and preservatives!
(talk about dying of "unnatural causes"!)

On that note, most foods already contain sodium. The body requires 2-3 times as much **potassium** as it does sodium. Most potassium comes from fresh fruit and vegetables. Salt is mainly used for preservation, and fluid balance, especially in pregnant women to replace fluids either for the fetus or in breast milk. Potassium promotes healthy growth. Calcium promotes contracting(tightening) of muscles, and magnesium promotes the relaxing of muscles and nerves. Too much calcium leads to kidney and gall stones, which apparently are extremely painful, and also calcifying of joints, a cause of arthritis.

1) Fat, Sick & Starved People

In spite of our wealth and advanced healthcare system, the United States is one of the sickest countries in the world.
Dead pharmaceutical drugs cannot overcome the effect of the Standard American Diet (SAD) on the human body and mind. As one doctor reputedly said, "No human is a perfect specimen."
Obesity has at least two causes: 1) food, and 2) slow metabolism (hypothyroidism).
Diabetes has 2 causes: 1) autoimmune insulin problems {"juvenile"}, 2) food {"diabetes Type 2"}
Illness has multiple causes: 1) diet, 2) environmental toxins/viruses & bacteria, 3) foodborne illness {food improperly handled, uncooked or under-cooked meat or seafood, out-dated or spoiled food, poor personal hygiene/cleanliness}, 4) genetics/DNA
Starvation: lack of or less-than appropriate food intake.
Malnutrition: less-than-appropriate food intake, or lack of nutrition, whether by food shortage, or low-nutrient foods, including junk foods. (also high-calorie low-nutrient foods)
The assumption is that if we were wealthier, we could afford better food. There are some very wealthy people who still eat, drink (and smoke) lots of junk. They have a "don't know, don't care" attitude. There are others who, with more money, invest it in high-quality foods, which naturally increase their health. Then there are those who, no matter how much money they make, invest it in high-quality foods as a habit, not just as a "luxury". But, the truth is, as "weird" as healthy food may seem, or look, or taste, it STILL generally keeps you healthier, and this saves you more money from not having to go to the doctor's office for this, that and the other. Most of us will say with a certain amount of accuracy, that doctors "live off of" people's sickness, while they do all they can to keep themselves healthy. Is it because they have all that money to spend? Or because they are "in control", or have "advanced knowledge", & treating the rest of us as paeans who don't know anything? Well, as human beings, we ALL have the freedom, and the right to choose. We choose good or bad food, good or bad activities, good or bad companions. There is a proverb saying your friends can be good for you, or they can destroy you, whether they are wise, or foolish.
People get drunk, or addicted to drugs, or any other vice, often (but not always) because they were associating with "foolish companions", or else had no purpose in life, or "too much time on their hands." Newsflash: "Ignorance is bliss" only lasts so long, before you end up in the hospital. And while doctors may "know" more, generally, about the human body, YOU know MORE about YOUR body than the doctor does. You know what affects it, its eccentricities, quirks, complaints, etc. Your doctor would have to talk with you or "check you out" for such a long period of time that you would probably go bankrupt from that one appointment. You also have the right to do your own research into alternative health practices, even healthier diets (acupuncture and homeopathy are not the only alternative health practices!). The book, <u>Prescription for Nutritional Healing</u> is one of a few excellent books for learning about herbal/natural remedies, foods that have a healing effect on certain illnesses, etc. Let me put it this way: for the cost of a heart surgery, ($30,000 on low end) you could make 450, $75 grocery trips for fruits, vegetables and healthy grains. Isn't that a lot cheaper than surgery? Plus, you wouldn't be in debt to the grocery store, you could buy the food **whenever** you wanted. Plus, you don't have to have health insurance to buy groceries, and that means you don't have to make an insurance "claim" to buy groceries. Granted, with all this food, some people need recipes to make meals, because it is beneficial to have good recipes for all that food you buy. Restaurant food and store-bought food has its pros and cons…sometimes it has more(or less) "stuff" than you want, which you can avoid by making your meals at home from fresh wholesome ingredients. Also, if you're creative enough, you can study the "restaurant food" and make your own version, according to YOUR diet, instead of their "standards" or franchise rules.
It's been said that those who do not govern themselves will be governed by tyrants.
The objective here is to eat the foods that will help you avoid expensive doctors and hospitals.

2) Balanced Alternatives

"The Usual" food:	**Alternatives:**
steaks, chicken, pork, burgers, shrimp	bean burgers, etc.
spinach-artichoke dip (usually with cheese)	non-dairy meltable cheese(available)
brownies and many other desserts (white flour/sugar)	gluten-free flour, brown sugar/dates
baked beans with pork fat	beans, onions, herbs/spices, avocado
shakes and beverages	whole-food smoothies
beer, liquor and wine	apple cider vinegar, lemon juice, etc.
quesadillas	tortillas with non-dairy cheese, etc.
cheesecake	Tofutti, soaked nuts~~, coconut
breads	gluten-free breads
candy/candy bars	fresh fruit, plain nuts, dark non-dairy chocolate
snack foods	non-fried, gluten-free/dairy-free/junk-free foods
grilled foods	sauteed/steamed foods
milk in so many chocolates	non-dairy milk (several available)
white rice	brown rice, other whole grains
wheat in soy sauce	non-fermented soy sauce, Bragg's Liquid Aminos
fully or partially hydrogenated peanut butter	plain ol' peanut butter, other nut butters
artificially-colored tortilla chips	chips from whole-grain flour
artificial color in wasabi sauce	real wasabi horseradish
eggs in horseradish and honey-mustard sauce	turmeric, real mustard flour, etc.
white sugar on brownies	Stevia, date sugar, etc.
pasta in minestrone	gluten-free pasta or vegetable pasta
beef in chili	buckwheat, cumin, coriander
salad dressings	wholesome ingredients, healthy oils
sauces	wholesome ingredients, healthy oils/fats
wheat flour in foods that shouldn't have wheat	several gluten-free thickeners available
gravies	corn starch,etc.

3) Piecemeal Healthy Foods

Salad bars
"vegan" or "gluten-free" options, instead of both
Salads
cornbread muffins (corn-wheat blend, typically)
gluten-free OR dairy-free pizzas, rarely both
gluten-free flour containing white rice flour(???)
"organic natural flavors"??
Chili with cheese(since when do Mexicans specialize in cheese??)
gluten-free soup or foods with dairy (both gluten and dairy have similar stifling effects on digestion)
restaurant house salad topped with cheese, as a standard
Mexican food with cheese. (nachos, tacos, refried beans, etc.)

4) Junk in Food

Processed Ingredient	Food/Substance/explanation:
refined flours	typically wheat, white rice
white rice	is there any "whole-grain white rice"?
artificial colorings	Blue & Yellow, Yellow Lake, Red, Blue, etc.)
artificial flavorings	
artificial preservatives	Monosodium Glutamate, etc.
unripe foods	(white cranberries, etc.)
white sugar, powdered or granulated	
agricultural chemicals	[ad nauseum] (will not list at the "risk" of getting sued)
hominy	lye (belongs in soap, not food)
high fructose corn syrup	you never leave the table satisfied
sodium nitrates, nitrites	would you like more "red" with your ham and bacon?
modified food starch	can contain wheat and other stuff (that's why it's so cheap!)

5) Monopoly of Certain Foods

1. Wheat, dairy, meat, corn, sorghum, soybeans. Few of any of these foods have Vitamin C, except soybeans and maybe corn.
2. At least one [soy] is a complete protein (that we know of), in spite of its presumed high-estrogen content.
3. All of these have been genetically modified to the seed "manufacturer's" pleasing.

4. Livestock require many thousands of gallons of water in cleaning up after them, whether manure, or their bloody, bacteria-ridden contaminating body parts, and also take several hours, not to mention countless gallons of water to thaw out in the kitchen before use.

6) Politics & Celebrities

Bureaucrats

USDA	United States Dept. of Agriculture	Covers: animals, plants, food safety, sanitation
ADA	American Dairy Association	Sales of dairy cows, milk, cheese, butter, etc.
AMA	American Medical Association	the "gods" of the "health care" industry
USRDA	US Recommended Dietary Allowance	Minimal nutrition to keep us basically alive
FDA	Food & Drug Administration (who spend more time on drugs than on real food) hint hint	
EPA	Environmental Protection Agency	

etc., etc.

"Good" celebrities:

David Wolfe (famous for promoting the RAW food lifestyle)
several RAW/VEGAN food athletes (football, boxing, etc.) [using Garden of Life products]
Roxanne Klein: former restaurateur of "Roxanne's", a raw restaurant formerly in California
Dr. Ann Wigmore, Hippocrates Institute, Creative Health Institute
Jordan Rubin/Garden of Life products, Raw/Organic foods, author of <u>The Raw Truth</u>
(see Title page and Suggested Reads for others)
Nomi Shannon: rawfoods.com chef
et al....

7) Conventional vs. Healthy

Conventional
steakhouses
fast-food
Italian restaurants
Pizza restaurants
Mexican restaurants
Hotel kitchens
"continental breakfast"

Definition: the omnivorous "eat anything, pay for it later" philosophy
motivation: lust, appearance, peer pressure, status quo, tradition
"fast" (as in, fried and/or grilled and ready to eat in under 10 minutes, maybe!)
heavy on bread, pasta & cheese (over-fed & under-nourished)
heavy on dough & cheese, usually pasta
white flour tortillas, cheese, sour cream
depends on which hotel chain. Some have "Midwestern", some have gourmet
Danishes, dry cereal?, fresh fruit?, muffins, eggs,meat,biscuits?,hashbrowns?
Easy & cheaper NOW, expensive later! (pay me now or pay me later)

Healthy
salad bar (typical)
garden produce
orchard produce
sea vegetables

Definition: selective "eat to live, to benefit body & mind, without guilt"
motivation: high value of self, self-education, despising medical costs
lettuce,greens,broccoli,radish,cucumber,tomato,olive,onion,bean,mushroom
anything that grows in the soil and is edible by and **safe** for humans(see list)
nuts,pears,apples,peaches,cherries,apricots,mangoes,bananas, citrus, etc.
kombu(similar to kelp), dulse,wakame, arame, kelp, nori(sushi wrap), etc.

organic vs. natural

"natural" and "organic" can have similar definitions, but just because white sugar is "organic" does not mean it's natural. Pressure-treated wood from an organic tree is not natural.
"organic" is a complex process of fertilization and crop maintenance which does not involve any non-organic pesticides, herbicides or fungicides, often using "green manure" (vetch, red clover, alfalfa,etc.) that enriches the soil with nitrogen and various valuable minerals and nutrients.To be "certified organic," crops must have been grown 3 years or more without mentioned agricultural chemicals. Any animal fertilizers must be from a certified organic source, thus there is a lot of paperwork and tracking.
Natural: nothing added, nothing subtracted, i.e. fresh picked from the garden
 (some food manufacturers apparently have their own definition of natural)
a.k.a. "au naturel" (French)
On the other hand: manure may be "natural" and "organic" but it SURE is not edible or safe for human consumption!! This is why, if you are planning to use manure for fertilizing, it must be added at least **3 months before** seeding to a vegetable garden at a ratio of 1 ton per hectare (works out to about 5-10 pounds for a 6 foot diameter garden). For flower gardens this rule does not apply unless you plan to use the flowers for eating. The amount is standard, as too much nitrogen (fertilizer in manure) will do more harm than good to your soil and plants, and will end up "burning" them, which typically turns the plants an ugly dead brown.

8) Nutrition--Animal-based food

	Qty.	Chol.	Cals.	g Prot.	g Sodium	g Fat	g S.Fat	g Fiber	B1	B2	B6	B12	18mg Iron	Vit. C	(A_RE) Vit. A
beef, ground, fried, well, lean	3 oz.	81	235	24	74	15	5.9	0	0.05	0.2	0.3	2.2	2.1	0	0
beef, ribeye steak, broiled lean	3 oz.	68	191	24	0	10	4	0	0.08	0.19	0.34	2.8	2.2	0	0
Beef Bologna	1 pc	13	72	3	226	7	2.8	0	0.01	0.02	0.04	0.3	0.4	5	0
butter, rgular salted	1 cup	497	1627	2	1877	184	115	0	0.01	0.08	0.01	0.3	0.4	0	1711
cheese, colby, shredded	1 cup	107	445	27	683	36	22.8	0	0.02	0.42	0.09	0.93	0.9	0	311
Cheese, cheddar, shredded	1 cup	119	455	28	702	37	23.8	0	0.03	0.42	0.08	0.94	0.8	0	342
cheese, Monterey Jack, shred	1 cup	101	421	28	606	34	21.6	0	0.02	0.44	0.09	0.93	0.8	0	286
cheese, mozzarella, shredded	1 cup	+++	318	22	421	24	14.9	0	0.02	0.28	0.10	0.74	0.2	0	272
cheese, parmesan, grated	1 cup	79	456	42	1861	30	19.1	0	0.0	0.4	0.1	1.4	1	0	173
Cheese, Brie, sliced	1 cup	144	481	30	906	40	25.1	0	0.10	0.75	0.34	2.4	0.7	0	262
Cheese, Feta, shredded	1 cup	219	649	35	2745	52	36.7	0	0.38	2.08	1.04	4.2	1.6	0	315
chicken, breast w/skin, roasted	1 ea.	82	193	29	70	8	2.2	0	0.06	0.12	0.55	0.31	1.1	0	26
cream cheese	1 cup	255	810	18	687	81	51	0	0.0	0.5	0.1	1	2.8	0	1013
fish, catfish, breaded fried fillet	1 ea.	70	199	16	244	12	2.9	0.4	0.06	0.12	0.16	1.65	1.2	0	7
fish, cod, Pacific, baked/broiled	1 fillet	42	94	21	82	1	0.1	0	0.02	0.05	0.42	0.94	0.3	3	9
fish, salmon, sockeye, baked/brl	1 fillet	135	335	42	102	17	3	0	0.33	0.26	0.34	8.99	0.90	0	98
milk, 2%	1 cup	18	121	8	122	5	2.9	0	0.10	0.40	0.10	0.89	0.1	2	139
Milk, nonfat skim	1 cup	4	86	8	0	0	0.3	0	0.09	0.34	0.10	0.93	0.1	2	149
Milk, whole, 3.3% fat	1 cup	33	150	8	120	8	5.2	0	0.09	0.40	0.10	0.87	0.1	2	76
Bacon, cooked, regular	3 pcs	16	109	6	303	9	3.3	0	0.13	0.05	0.05	0.3	0.3	6	0
Ham, whole roasted lean & fat	1 cup	87	340	30	1661	24	8.4	0	0.84	0.31	0.53	0.90	1.2	0	0
Sausage, pepperoni, pork/beef	4 pcs	17	109	5	449	10	3.5	0.00	0.07	0.06	0.06	0.55	0.3	0.00	0.00
Sausage, Pork, Italian link, ck'd	1 ea.	52	216	13	618	17	6.1	0	0.42	0.16	0.22	0.88	1	1	0
Sausage, turkey, smoked	1 oz	19	55	4	219	4	1.3	0	0.02	0.06	0.06	0.56	0.4	0.00	0.00
Sausage, kielbasa (26 grams)	1 pc	17	81	3	280	7	2.6	0	0.06	0.06	0.05	0.42	0.4	5	0
Burger King, Whopper w/chz	1 ea.	115	730	33	1350	46	16	3	0.34	0.48	0.33	0	4.5	9	150
McDonalds cheeseburger	1 ea.		319	15	768	13	5.6	1.9	0.33	0.31	0.15	1.2	2.7	2	

For reference:
raw whole carrot, Vit. A=2025

9) Health-related Surgeries $$K

Name of surgery	Low $	High $	Average $
Angioplasty	$ 16,000	$ 61,000	
appendectomy	$ 5,000	$ 14,000	
cancer/tumor			$ 40,000
Cataract	$ 3,700	$ 8,000	
colorectomy(colon)			$ 14,000
gall bladder			$ 14,000
heart bypass	$ 47,000	$ 151,000	
Hip prosthesis	$ 11,000	$ 25,000	
hip replacement	$ 16,000	$ 53,000	
Knee replacement	$ 25,000	$ 51,000	
liver replacement			$20,000
normal child delivery	$ 10,000	$ 17,000	
stroke/aneurysm			$30,000+

10) Countless diseases from SAD

Standard **A**merican **D**iet		Physiological
Illness	**Affected**	**Response**
Diabetes	Insulin, pancreas	fainting, etc.
Stroke	brain, circulatory system	brain problems, loss of speech, motion, nerve impulses
Gall stones	Gall bladder, excess of calcium	pain
Kidney stones	Kidneys, urethra, urinary tract	pain
cardiac arrest	heart, blood vessels, brain, life	chest pain, collapse, die, heart stops, brain lacks oxygen
arthritis, gout	joints (fingers, feet, knees, wrist, etc.)	painful joints and movement, swelling around joints
atherosclerosis	blood vessels--excess cholesterol	eventual cardiac arrest, plaque buildup, slows blood flow
cirrhosis	liver--alcohol, malnutrition	fatigue, weight loss, vomiting, weakness, skin yellowing
Colitis, IBS, etc.	intestines--clogged w/fiberless junk	constipation, auto-intoxication, bloating, pain, nausea, etc.

11) Healthy Foods, Big Appetites

Most of the "healthy" food you see is contained in a 10-30 cubic inch space on a plate(2-3 inches), and you're thinking, "That's all????" I've seen what athletes can eat (they can really put it down!). I've often wondered, if athletes ate healthy, what would their plate look like? If they were eating at a buffet restaurant, they would easily wolf down 2-3 or more plates of food. And then there are the vegan/raw athletes. We're probably talking 2-3 "Burrito bowls" at Chipotle or something like that. Then you get these "raw cuisine schools" and they spend so much time making the plate look "pretty" that there's not much time spent in making it SATISFYING. Let's say if someone at a hotel banquet is getting a vegan meal, and everyone else is getting, let's say, chicken marsala with broccoli and rice pilaf, do you think they'll be satisfied with a 3" pretty salad? I don't think so. As a banquet cook, I know what I'm talking about. And that's not even an athlete. Or, maybe there is a concert pianist--they spend lots of energy playing all that music, they most likely work up an appetite! Maybe it's different from guys to girls, but still. Calories have to be replaced, and let's hope it's nutrient-dense calories, because anything less would be a joke, and clog up their joints. A concert pianist with arthritis?? Not on your life. Concert musician, athlete, gymnast, whatever; they're probably careful about what they eat, to a certain extent; well, maybe except for athletes in general. Carbohydrates are the tricky part. Bagels and sugar-loaded pastries? Maybe baseball players and football players. But everyone has their own preferences and dislikes, or, one man's trash is another man's treasure. Then you have allergies coming into the picture, which makes the road all that much narrower. What can you replace bagels and cream cheese with? Good question. Oatmeal? Cooked hot cereal? Fruit is good but the water content may not maintain a "full" feeling. Thoughts to ponder. This is why nutrition is one of the most detail-oriented professions, because every person has a little bit different dietary, chemical and immune composition. Then again, fake food is always fake food, and does more good for your doctor than it does for you. Think about it.

12) Calories and Sugars 101

white-sugar-loaded "dessert" **equals =**	high-glycemic=sugar crash=insulin emergency=diabetes
high calories **does not equal**	high nutrition or energy capacity
invert sugars in "factory" foods **vs.**	complex sugars naturally in whole foods
low glycemic foods=long-lasting energy--	fruits, vegetables, whole sprouted or raw legumes, nuts, seeds
3 most important monosaccharides in diet	fructose, glucose, galactose
Glucose: monosaccharide	primary form of carbo-hydrate used to produce body fuel/energy (a.k.a. blood sugar)
	Glucose is also produced by photosynthesis in plants
	Insulin promotes storage of glucose in liver as glycogen and lesser so as fat. Insulin stimulates glucose uptake by muscle
Sucrose: disaccharide	formed by connecting glucose to fructose.
	Found in sugar cane, sugar beets, honey & maple syrup
	Only sweetener that can officially be called "Sugar" on labels commonly known as regular white table sugar.
Galactose: part of lactose, or milk sugar	
Maltose:	2 glucose molecules joined together(starch broken)
Fructose: monosaccharide	sweeter than glucose, found in fruits and vegetables
	more than half of the sugar in honey
Glycogen:	carbohydrate storage in animals; made of
	highly branched glucose molecule chains, breaking down to glucose when needed.
Polysaccharides:	glycogen in animals, plant starch & fiber
Oligosaccharides:	short chain carbs with 3-10 sugar units,
	often found in beans and legumes (raffinose, starchyose)
Honey:	bees collect, turn sucrose into fructose & glucose
Blackstrap molasses:	refined sucrose from sugar cane or sugar beets

13) Well-being vs. Healthcare

Honest questions to make you THINK--HEALTH ECONOMICS

Nutritionist	vs doctor/hospital	doctors are not trained in nutrition, only anatomy & physiology
fruits & vegetables	vs pharmaceutical	no side effects vs. drug side effects related or unrelated to illness
massage therapist	vs massage chair	chair costs more for the sake of 24/7/365 convenience, robotic "fingers"
Organic	vs GMO	what separates ethical GMO from unethical GMO?
food & supplements	vs vaccines	nutrient-rich food, or the medical system's dangerous chemicals?

Drug vs. Food Remedy Chart

DRUG NAME	HEALTH CLAIM	HERB/FOOD REMEDY
Symbicort	COPD(Cardiopulmonary disease)	legumes,nuts,avocado,flax,etc.
Lipitor	cholesterol-lowering	Omega-3 oils(flax,walnut,etc.)
fluconasol	nasal congestion	nut milks, onions,garlic,pepper

(the following info from "*taste for life*" magazine, Sept. 2003,pp 16-19)

Valium	anxiety	kava, chamomile, lavender
Celebrex	arthritis	turmeric, cherries
Hytrin	BPH(Benign Prostatic Hypertrophy)	saw palmetto,pumpkin seed
Prosgar	BPH	evening primrose oil
Cognex	dementia	ginkgo biloba,gotu kola,lecithin
Allopurinol	gout	celery seed, dark cherries
Prozac	PMS, depression, social anxiety	evening primrose oil, kava
verapamil	heart disease	hawthorn berry
zocor	high cholesterol	garlic, flax, nuts, legumes

Animal-based and processed foods vs. natural plant-based foods, and FIBER:
It has been biologically documented that carnivores have shorter intestines than plant-
to the rapidly-decaying properties of dead foods. This is why animal foods require so n
The shorter the tunnel, the quicker the stuff gets out, preventing excessive putrefaction
eating animal's intestine is longer, to absorb as many nutrients as possible from the di
Putrefaction leads to auto-intoxication, eventually leading to death. For an animal, no
unique life and purpose lost.

DFC

Drug vs. Food Remedy Chart

AVOID
red meat,dairy,margarine
animal foods, trans-fats
dairy foods,ragweed flowers

guilty pleasures,excess stress
white flour/sugar/grains
high-estrogen foods, etc.

"white" flour/sugar/grains
processed flour & sugar
wheat, processed sugar
high-fat processed foods
high-fat processed foods

eating animals. This is due
much salt & preservation.
. On the other hand, a plant-
gested plant material.
big deal. For a human, a

DFC

Nutrition--Fruits

Nutrients -- 100grams edible portion

Fruit	1 oz = 28.35 grams Typical Weight(g)	Individual Qty per 100g	(cups) volume per 100g	Calories	g Protein
Apple, raw w/skin 3"	215	0.47		59	0.19
Apricot, fresh	84			48	1.4
Apricot, dried, unsulph.	20			260	5
Banana, raw	200	0.5		80	1.3
Blackberry, raw	8			52	0.72
Blueberry, raw	6	70		56	0.67
Boysenberry, raw	10			50	1.1
Cherry, Acerola,raw	5			32	0.4
Cherry, Common,raw sweet	6	16	3/4 cup	72	1.2
Cherry,Common,raw sour	2.7	37	3/4 cup	50	1
Cranberry, raw	10			49	0.39
Currant, raw black	5			63	1.4
Currant, raw red/white	5			56	1.4
Date, dried	35			274-293	1.7-3.9
Elderberry, raw	4			73	0.66
Feijoa, raw	56			49	1.24
Fig, dried	20	5		274	4.3
Grape,raw Concord	10			63	0.63
Raisin,raw brown seedless	5		5/8 cup	300	3.22
Grapefruit,fresh fruit	300			40	0.75
Guava,raw	65			42	1
Kiwi fruit,raw	67	1.5		66	0.79
Kumquat,raw	28			274	3.8
Lemon,raw w/o peel	104	0.96		29	1.1
Lime,raw	84			30	0.09
Loganberry,raw	20			55	1.52
Mango,raw	308			62	0.38
Melon,Cantaloupe,raw	1344			35	0.88
Melon,Honeydew,raw	2016			35	0.46
Melon,Casaba,raw	2130			26	0.9
Mulberry,raw	10			43	1.44
Nectarine,raw	180			49	0.94
Orange,raw	280			49	1
Tangerine,raw(mandarin)	88	1.14		46	0.8
Papaya,raw,regular	504			24	0.21
Peach,raw	168			43	0.7
Pear,raw	224			59	0.39
Pear,Asian,raw	196			42	0.5
Persimmon,raw American	170			127	0.8
Pineapple,raw, standard	1568	1/16 pineapple		49	0.39
Plum,raw Damson	112			66	0.5
Prune,raw dried	112			239	2.61
Raspberry,raw fruit	10			49	0.91
Raspberry,leaves,dried	1		4 cups	275	11.3
Rhubarb,raw(12" stalk)	79	1 1/4 stalks	7/8 cup	21	0.9
Strawberry,raw	70			30	0.61
Tamarind,raw pod	28			172	3.1
Tomatillo,raw	84			32	0.42
Watermelon,raw	5376			32	0.62

Miscellaneous Fruit: **Typical weight**

star fruit	9 oz (255g)
quince	7 oz (198g)
pepino melon	5 oz (142g)
kiwano melon	10 oz (284g)
pomegranate	12 oz (340g)

Nutrition--Fruits

Fruit	g Fat	35 g Fiber	10,000IU A (IU)	50mg B1	50mg B2	100mg B3 Niacin	100mg Pant.Acid	50mg B6
Apple, raw w/skin 3"	0.36	0.77	53	0.017	0.014	0.077	0.061	0.048
Apricot, fresh	0.39	0.6	2612	0.03	0.04	0.6	0.24	0.054
Apricot, dried, unsulph.	0.5	3	10900	0.01	0.16	3.3		
Banana, raw	0.2	0.6		0.29	0.055	0.8	0.26	0.578
Blackberry, raw	0.39	4.1	165	0.03	0.04	0.4	0.24	0.058
Blueberry, raw	0.38	1.3	100	0.048	0.05	0.359	0.093	0.036
Boysenberry, raw	0.26	2.7	67	0.053	0.037	0.4	0.25	0.056
Cherry, Acerola,raw	0.3	0.4	767	0.02	0.06	0.359	0.3	0.009
Cherry, Common,raw sweet	0.96	0.4	214	0.05	0.06	0.767	0.127	0.036
Cherry,Common,raw sour	0.3	0.2	1283	0.03	0.04	0.4	0.143	0.044
Cranberry, raw	0.2	1.2	46	0.03	0.02	0.4	0.219	0.065
Currant, raw black	0.41	2.4	230	0.05	0.05	0.4	0.398	0.066
Currant, raw red/white	0.2	3.4	120	0.04	0.05	0.1	0.064	0.07
Date, dried	.1-1.2	2.0-8.5	50	0.06	0.13	0.3	0.78	0.192
Elderberry, raw	0.5	7	600	0.07	0.06	0.1	0.14	0.23
Feijoa, raw	0.78			0.008	0.032	1.8	0.228	0.05
Fig, dried	1.3	5.6	100	0.071	0.088	0.5	0.435	0.224
Grape,raw Concord	0.35	0.76	100	0.092	0.057	0.289	0.024	0.11
Raisin,raw brown seedless	0.46	1.28	8	0.156	0.088	0.694	0.045	0.249
Grapefruit,fresh fruit	0.13	.14-.77	440	0.045	0.015	0.3	0.283	0.042
Guava,raw	0.3	2.8-5.5	450	0.046	0.035	0.818	0.15	0.143
Kiwi fruit,raw	0.25	1.1	175	0.02	0.05	0.22		
Kumquat,raw	0.4	3.7	2530	0.35	0.4	0.8		
Lemon,raw w/o peel	0.3	0.4	29	0.04	0.02	0.5	0.19	0.08
Lime,raw	0.1	.1-.5	10	0.044	0.016		0.217	
Loganberry,raw	0.31	3	35	0.05	0.034	0.1	0.244	0.065
Mango,raw	0.41	.85-1.06	3894	0.045	0.046	0.19	0.16	0.134
Melon,Cantaloupe,raw	0.28	0.36	3224	0.036	0.021	0.84	0.128	0.115
Melon,Honeydew,raw	0.1	0.6	40	0.077	0.018	0.35	0.207	0.059
Melon,Casaba,raw	0.1	0.5	30	0.06	0.02	0.574		
Mulberry,raw	0.39	0.96	25	0.029	0.101	0.6		
Nectarine,raw	0.46	0.4	736	0.017	0.041	0.4	0.158	0.025
Orange,raw	0.2	0.5	200	0.1	0.04	0.62	0.25	0.06
Tangerine,raw(mandarin)	0.2	0.5	420	0.105	0.022	0.99	0.2	0.067
Papaya,raw,regular	0.5	.5-1.3	2014	0.029	0.041	0.4	0.218	0.019
Peach,raw	0.09	0.64	535	0.017	0.041	0.16	0.17	0.018
Pear,raw	0.4	1.4	20	0.02	0.04	0.34	0.07	0.018
Pear,Asian,raw	0.23			0.009	0.01	0.99	0.07	0.022
Persimmon,raw American	0.4	1.5				0.1		
Pineapple,raw, standard	0.43	.3-.6	23	0.098	0.025	0.219	0.16	0.09
Plum,raw Damson	0.01	0.4	300	0.08	0.03			0.05
Prune,raw dried	0.52	2.04	1987	0.081	0.162	0.19		0.264
Raspberry,raw fruit	0.55	3	130	0.03	0.09	0.5	0.24	0.057
Raspberry,leaves,dried	1.7	8.2	18963	0.34		1.961		
Rhubarb,raw(12" stalk)	0.2	0.7	130	0.03	0.09	0.9	0.24	0.057
Strawberry,raw	0.37	0.53	27	0.02	0.066	38.2	0.34	0.059
Tamarind,raw pod	0.1	5.6	22	0.29	0.11	0.9	0.143	0.066
Tomatillo,raw	0.6	.6-1.7	80	0.075	0.035	0.23	0.15	0.056
Watermelon,raw	0.43	0.3	366	0.08	0.02	1.2	0.212	0.144

Nutrition--Fruits

Fruit	(mcg) 800mcg Folic Acid	3000mg Vitamin C	600IU 40 IU=1 mcg Vitamin E	1500 mg Calcium	3mg Copper
Apple, raw w/skin 3"	2.8	5.7	0.59	7	0.031
Apricot, fresh	8.6	10		14	0.089
Apricot, dried, unsulph.		12		67	
Banana, raw	19.1	18	0.27	8	0.104
Blackberry, raw		21	0.6	32	0.14
Blueberry, raw	6.4	13		6	0.061
Boysenberry, raw	63.3	3.1		27	0.08
Cherry, Acerola,raw		1677.6		12	
Cherry, Common,raw sweet	4.2	7		15	0.095
Cherry,Common,raw sour	7.5	10	0.13	16	0.104
Cranberry, raw	1.7	13.5		7	0.058
Currant, raw black		181	1	55	0.086
Currant, raw red/white		41	0.1	33	0.107
Date, dried	2.6			81	0.288
Elderberry, raw		36		38	
Feijoa, raw	38	31		11	0.055
Fig, dried	7.5	0.8		126	0.313
Grape,raw Concord	3.9	4		14	0.04
Raisin,raw brown seedless	3.3	3.3		49	0.309
Grapefruit,fresh fruit	10.2	43	0.25	20	0.047
Guava,raw		300		13	0.103
Kiwi fruit,raw		90		20	
Kumquat,raw		151		266	0.107
Lemon,raw w/o peel	10.6	53		26	0.037
Lime,raw	8.2	39		17	0.065
Loganberry,raw	25.7	15.3		26	0.117
Mango,raw		87	1.12	9	0.11
Melon,Cantaloupe,raw	17	42.2	0.14	11	0.042
Melon,Honeydew,raw		24.8		6	0.041
Melon,Casaba,raw		16		5	
Mulberry,raw		36.4		39	
Nectarine,raw	3.7	5.4		5	0.073
Orange,raw	30.3	52	0.24	40	0.045
Tangerine,raw(mandarin)	20.4	31		40	0.028
Papaya,raw,regular		53		25	0.016
Peach,raw	3.4	6.6		5	0.068
Pear,raw	7.3	4	0.5	11	0.113
Pear,Asian,raw	8	2.5		4	0.05
Persimmon,raw American		66		27	
Pineapple,raw, standard	10.6	42	0.1	21	0.11
Plum,raw Damson				18	
Prune,raw dried		3.3		51	
Raspberry,raw fruit		25	0.3	22	0.074
Raspberry,leaves,dried		367		1210	
Rhubarb,raw(12" stalk)		25	0.3	86	0.074
Strawberry,raw	17.7	56.7	0.12	14	0.049
Tamarind,raw pod		1.8		110	
Tomatillo,raw	7	3		8	0.079
Watermelon,raw	2.2	9.6		8	0.032

Nutrition--Fruits

Fruit	18mg Iron	1000mg Magnesium	10mg Manganese	Fruit	600mg Phosphorus	2000mg Potass.
Apple, raw w/skin 3"	0.18	5	0.023	Apple, raw w/skin 3"	7	115
Apricot, fresh	0.54	8	0.079	Apricot, fresh	19	296
Apricot, dried, unsulph.	5.5			Apricot, dried, unsulph.	108	979
Banana, raw	0.9	29	0.152	Banana, raw	33	396
Blackberry, raw	0.57	20	1.291	Blackberry, raw	21	196
Blueberry, raw	0.17	5	0.282	Blueberry, raw	10	89
Boysenberry, raw	0.85	16	0.547	Boysenberry, raw	27	139
Cherry, Acerola,raw	0.2	18		Cherry, Acerola,raw	11	146
Cherry, Common,raw sweet	0.39	11	0.092	Cherry, Common,raw swt	19	224
Cherry,Common,raw sour	0.32	9	0.112	Cherry,Common,raw sour	15	173
Cranberry, raw	0.2	5	0.157	Cranberry, raw	9	71
Currant, raw black	1.54	24	0.256	Currant, raw black	59	322
Currant, raw red/white	1	13	0.186	Currant, raw red/white	44	275
Date, dried	8	35	0.298	Date, dried	83	648
Elderberry, raw	1.6			Elderberry, raw	39	280
Feijoa, raw	0.065	8.5	0.085	Feijoa, raw	15	161
Fig, dried	3	59	0.388	Fig, dried	77	640
Grape,raw Concord	0.29	5	0.718	Grape,raw Concord	10	191
Raisin,raw brown seedless	2.08	33	0.308	Raisin,raw brown seedless	97	751
Grapefruit,fresh fruit	0.4	8	0.012	Grapefruit,fresh fruit	31	137
Guava,raw	0.5	17	0.144	Guava,raw	23	284
Kiwi fruit,raw	0.51	30		Kiwi fruit,raw	52	332
Kumquat,raw	1.7	13	0.086	Kumquat,raw	97	995
Lemon,raw w/o peel	0.6			Lemon,raw w/o peel	16	138
Lime,raw	0.25			Lime,raw	15	102
Loganberry,raw	0.64	21	1.247	Loganberry,raw	26	145
Mango,raw	0.4	9	0.027	Mango,raw	11	156
Melon,Cantaloupe,raw	0.21	11	0.047	Melon,Cantaloupe,raw	17	309
Melon,Honeydew,raw	0.07	7	0.018	Melon,Honeydew,raw	10	271
Melon,Casaba,raw	0.4	8		Melon,Casaba,raw	7	210
Mulberry,raw	1.85	18		Mulberry,raw	38	194
Nectarine,raw	0.15	8	0.044	Nectarine,raw	16	212
Orange,raw	0.5	10	0.025	Orange,raw	19.5	195
Tangerine,raw(mandarin)	0.4	12	0.032	Tangerine,raw(mandarin)	18	126
Papaya,raw,regular	0.5	10	0.011	Papaya,raw,regular	13	257
Peach,raw	0.11	7	0.047	Peach,raw	12	197
Pear,raw	0.25	6	0.076	Pear,raw	11	125
Pear,Asian,raw		8	0.06	Pear,Asian,raw	11	121
Persimmon,raw American	2.5			Persimmon,raw American	26	310
Pineapple,raw, standard	0.27	14	1.649	Pineapple,raw, standard	8.5	113
Plum,raw Damson	0.5			Plum,raw Damson	17	299
Prune,raw dried	2.48			Prune,raw dried	79	745
Raspberry,raw fruit	0.57	18	1.013	Raspberry,raw fruit	12	152
Raspberry,leaves,dried	101	319	146	Raspberry,leaves,dried	234	1340
Rhubarb,raw(12" stalk)	0.22	12	1.013	Rhubarb,raw(12" stalk)	14	288
Strawberry,raw	0.38	10	0.29	Strawberry,raw	19	166
Tamarind,raw pod	5.0	92		Tamarind,raw pod	80	501
Tomatillo,raw	1.0	23	0.153	Tomatillo,raw	31	243
Watermelon,raw	0.17	11	0.037	Watermelon,raw	9	116

Nutrition--Fruits

Fruit	Sodium (mg)	Zinc 50mg
Apple, raw w/skin 3"	0	0.04
Apricot, fresh	1	0.26
Apricot, dried, unsulph.	26	
Banana, raw	1	0.16
Blackberry, raw	0	0.27
Blueberry, raw	6	0.11
Boysenberry, raw	1	0.22
Cherry, Acerola, raw	7	
Cherry, Common, raw sweet	0	0.06
Cherry, Common, raw sour	3	0.1
Cranberry, raw	1	0.13
Currant, raw black	2	0.27
Currant, raw red/white	1	0.23
Date, dried	3	0.29
Elderberry, raw		
Feijoa, raw	4	0.04
Fig, dried	22	0.51
Grape, raw Concord	2	0.04
Raisin, raw brown seedless	21	0.27
Grapefruit, fresh fruit	1	0.07
Guava, raw	3	0.23
Kiwi fruit, raw	5	
Kumquat, raw		0.08
Lemon, raw w/o peel		0.06
Lime, raw	2	0.11
Loganberry, raw	1	0.34
Mango, raw	2	0.04
Melon, Cantaloupe, raw	9	0.16
Melon, Honeydew, raw	1	
Melon, Casaba, raw	12	
Mulberry, raw	10	
Nectarine, raw	0	0.09
Orange, raw	1	0.07
Tangerine, raw (mandarin)	2	
Papaya, raw, regular	3	0.07
Peach, raw	0	0.14
Pear, raw		0.12
Pear, Asian, raw		0.02
Persimmon, raw American	1	
Pineapple, raw, standard	1.2	0.08
Plum, raw Damson	2	
Prune, raw dried	4	
Raspberry, raw fruit	0	0.46
Raspberry, leaves, dried	7.7	
Rhubarb, raw (12" stalk)	4	0.1
Strawberry, raw	1	0.13
Tamarind, raw pod	24	
Tomatillo, raw	0.4	0.22
Watermelon, raw	2	0.07

Nutrition--Grains

Nutrient Info per 100grams edible portion

Grain	2 Qty / 100g	(cups) volume / 100g	Calories	g Protein
Amaranth, raw whole grain			374	14.45
Amaranth, raw leaves			26	2.46
Buckwheat, raw whole grain			343	13.25
Buckwheat, whole grain dark flour			335	12.62
Corn, raw whole grain			365	9.42
Corn, whole grain meal			362	8.12
Corn, plain popcorn (uncooked)			386	12.7
Millet, raw whole grain		1/2 cup	378	11.02
Millet, cooked whole grain			119	3.51
Quinoa, raw whole grain	1/2 cup		374	13.1
Quinoa flour			354	10.4
Rice, long grain brown, cooked			111	2.58
Rice bran			316	13.35
Rice flour, brown rice			363	7.23
Wild rice, cooked			101	3.99
Sorghum, raw whole grain			339	11.3

Grain	Sodium	50mg Zinc
Amaranth, raw whole grain	21	3.18
Amaranth, raw leaves	20	0.9
Buckwheat, raw whole grain	1	2.4
Buckwheat, whole grain dark flour		3.12
Corn, raw whole grain	35	2.21
Corn, whole grain meal	35	1.82
Corn, plain popcorn (uncooked)	3	
Millet, raw whole grain	5	1.68
Millet, cooked whole grain	2	0.91
Quinoa, raw whole grain		3.3
Quinoa flour		
Rice, long grain brown, cooked	5	0.63
Rice bran	5	6.04
Rice flour, brown rice	8	2.45
Wild rice, cooked	3	1.34
Sorghum, raw whole grain		

Nutrition--Grains

Grain	g Fat	35 g Fiber	10,000IU Vit. A	50mg B1	50mg B2	100mg B3 Niacin	100mg Pant.Acid	50mg B6
Amaranth, raw whole grain	6.51	3.77		0.08	0.208	1.286	1.047	0.223
Amaranth, raw leaves	0.33	0.98	2917	0.027	0.158	0.658		
Buckwheat, raw whole grain	3.4	9.9		0.101	0.425	7.02		0.21
Buckwheat, whole grain dark flour	3.1	1.6		0.417	0.19	6.15	0.44	0.582
Corn, raw whole grain	4.74	2.9		0.385	0.201	3.627	0.424	0.622
Corn, whole grain meal	3.59	1.84	469	0.385	0.201	3.632	0.425	0.304
Corn, plain popcorn (uncooked)	5	2.2			0.12	2.2		
Millet, raw whole grain	4.22	1.03		0.42	0.29	4.72	0.848	0.384
Millet, cooked whole grain	1	0.36		0.106	0.082	1.33	0.171	0.108
Quinoa, raw whole grain	5.8			0.198	0.396	2.93		
Quinoa flour	4	3.8		0.19	0.24	0.7		
Rice, long grain brown, cooked	0.9	0.34		0.096	0.025	1.528	0.285	0.145
Rice bran	20.85	11.5		2.753	0.284	33.995	7.39	4.07
Rice flour, brown rice	2.78	1.29		0.443	0.08	6.34	1.59	0.736
Wild rice, cooked	0.34	0.33		0.052	0.087	1.287	0.154	0.135
Sorghum, raw whole grain	3.3	2.4		0.237	0.142	2.927		

Nutrition--Grains

	800mcg	300mcg	3g	40 IU=1 mcg 400IU	600IU	1500 mg
Grain	Folic Acid	B12	Vit. C	Vit. D	Vit. E	Calcium
Amaranth, raw whole grain	49		4.2			153
Amaranth, raw leaves	85.3		43.3			215
Buckwheat, raw whole grain	30					18
Buckwheat, whole grain dark flour	54					41
Corn, raw whole grain					0.49	7
Corn, whole grain meal						6
Corn, plain popcorn (uncooked)						11
Millet, raw whole grain					0.05	8
Millet, cooked whole grain						3
Quinoa, raw whole grain						60
Quinoa flour						94
Rice, long grain brown, cooked	4					10
Rice bran	63					57
Rice flour, brown rice	16					11
Wild rice, cooked	26					3
Sorghum, raw whole grain						28

	3mg	18mg	1g	10mg	600mg	2000mg
Grain	Copper	Iron	Mag	Manganese	Phosph	Potass.
Amaranth, raw whole grain	0.777	7.59	266	2.26	455	366
Amaranth, raw leaves	0.162	2.32	55		50	611
Buckwheat, raw whole grain	1.1	2.2	231	1.3	347	460
Buckwheat, whole grain dark flour	0.515	4.06	251	2.03	337	577
Corn, raw whole grain	0.314	2.71	127	0.485	210	287
Corn, whole grain meal	0.193	3.45	127	0.498	241	287
Corn, plain popcorn (uncooked)		2.7			281	
Millet, raw whole grain	0.75	3.01	114	1.632	285	195
Millet, cooked whole grain	0.161	0.63	44	0.272	100	62
Quinoa, raw whole grain	0.82	9.25	210		410	740
Quinoa flour		5.6			129	
Rice, long grain brown, cooked	0.1	0.42	43	0.905	83	43
Rice bran	0.728	18.54	781	14.21	1677	1485
Rice flour, brown rice	0.23	1.98	112	4.013	337	289
Wild rice, cooked	0.121	0.6	32	0.282	82	101
Sorghum, raw whole grain		4.4			287	350

per 100 grams edible portion

Legume	cups per 100g	Calories	g Protein	g Fat	35 g Fiber	10,000IU A
Aduki/Adzuki	1/2 cup + 1 tsp	128	7.52	0.1	2.02	6
Black-eyed pea	1/2 cup + 1 tsp	116	7.73	0.53	2.31	15
Chickpea/garbanzo	1/2 cup	164	8.86	2.59	2.5	27
Black bean		132	8.86	0.54	2.03	6
Pinto bean		137	8.21	0.52	3.02	2
Red bean		127	8.67	0.5	2.81	
French green lentils(lentil)	1/2 cup	116	9.02	0.38	2.76	8
Mung bean, sprouted raw		30	3.04	0.18	0.81	21
Peas		118	8.34	0.39	1.97	7
Soybean,mature,cooked		173	16.64	8.97	2.03	9
Soybean,sprouted raw		122	13.09	6.7	2.3	11

	50mg B1	50mg B2	100mg B3 Niacin	100mg Pant.Acid	50mg B6
Aduki/Adzuki	0.115	0.064	0.717		
Black-eyed pea	0.202	0.055	0.495	0.411	0.1
Chickpea/garbanzo	0.116	0.063	0.526	0.286	0.139
Black bean	0.244	0.059	0.505	0.242	0.069
Pinto bean	0.186	0.091	0.4	0.285	0.155
Red bean	0.16	0.058	0.578	0.22	0.12
French green lentils(lentil)	0.169	0.073	1.06	0.638	0.178
Mung bean, sprouted raw	0.084	0.124	0.749	0.38	0.088
Peas	0.19	0.056	0.89	0.595	0.048
Soybean,mature,cooked	0.155	0.285	0.399	0.179	0.234
Soybean,sprouted raw	0.34	0.118	1.148	0.929	0.176

		800mcg Folic Acid	3000mg Vitamin C	1500 mg Calcium	3mg Copper	18mg Iron
Aduki/Adzuki				28	0.298	2
Black-eyed pea		207.9	0.4	24	0.268	2.51
Chickpea/garbanzo		172	1.3	49	0.352	2.89
Black bean		148.8		27	0.209	2.1
Pinto bean		172	2.1	48	0.257	2.61
Red bean		129.6	1.2	28	0.242	2.94
French green lentils(lentil)	1/2 cup	180.8	1.5	19	0.251	3.33
Mung bean, sprouted raw		60.8	13.2	13	0.164	0.91
Peas		64.9	0.4	14	0.181	1.29
Soybean,mature,cooked		53.8	1.7	102	0.407	5.14
Soybean,sprouted raw		172	15.3	67	0.427	2.1

	1000mg Magnesium	10mg Manganese	600mg Phos	2000mg Potassium	50mg Zinc	Sodium
Aduki/Adzuki	52	0.573	168	532	1.77	8
Black-eyed pea	53	0.475	156	278	1.29	4
Chickpea/garbanzo	48	1.03	168	291	1.53	7
Black bean	70	0.444	140	355	1.12	1
Pinto bean	55	0.556	160	468	1.08	2
Red bean	45	0.477	142	403	1.07	2
French green lentils(lentil) 1/2 cup	36	0.494	180	369	1.27	2
Mung bean, sprouted raw	21	0.188	54	149	0.41	6
Peas	36	0.396	99	362	1	2
Soybean,mature,cooked	86	0.824	245	515	1.15	1
Soybean,sprouted raw	72	0.702	164	484	1.17	14

Nutrition--Nuts, Seeds & Oils

Nutrient Info per 100grams edible portion 2, 9

Item	(individual) Weight(g)	Qty / 100g	Volume per 100g (cups)	Calories	g Protein	g Fat	35 g Fiber
Alfalfa, sprouted raw				29	3.99	0.69	1.64
Alfalfa, dried				269	19.9	4.3	21
Almond, dried, unblanched		114		589	19.95	52.21	2.71
Brazil, dried, unblanched		24		656	14.34	66.22	2.29
Cashew, dry roasted				574	15.31	46.35	0.7
Chia seeds, dried(B2: 1 oz)				472	16.62	26.25	25.3
Flax seed, dried	3/4 cup = 110g			450	24	37	27.5
Hazelnut, Filbert, dried, unblanched			2/3 cup	632	13.04	62.64	3.8
Macadamia nut, dried				702	8.3	73.72	5.28
Olives, black, canned				98	0.91	8.3	
Olive oil(B2: 1 Tbsp)		125mL	1/2 cup	884	0	100	
Peanut oil, roasted(B2: 1 Tbsp)				581	26.35	49.3	5.33
Peanut, dry roasted	1/4 cup = 30g			571	25	50	7
Pecan, dried		50		667	7.75	67.64	1.6
Pine nut, dried(B2: 1 oz)				540	17	55	2
Pistachio, dried				577	20.58	48.39	1.88
Psyllium seed, dried				235	1.5	3.7	0.3
Pumpkin seed, dried		40/ tsp=1279	2/3 cup	541	24.54	45.85	2.22
Sesame seed, whole, dried			5/8 cup	573	17.73	49.67	4.6
Sunflower seed, dried	5/8 cup = 90g			570	22.78	49.57	4.16
Walnut, English dried	1/2 cup = 60g		3/4 cup	642	14.29	61.87	4.6
Walnut, Black dried				607	24.35	56.58	6.46
Watermelon seed, dried				557	28.33	47.37	3.04
Average				**522.5**	**15.9**	**46.2**	**6.4**

	10,000IU Vitamin A	50mg B1	50mg B2	100mg B3 Niacin	100mg Pant.Acid	50mg B6	800mcg Folate
Alfalfa, sprouted raw	155	0.076		0.481	0.563	0.034	36
Alfalfa, dried	24800	0.19		9.7			
Almond, dried, unblanched		0.211	0.28	3.361	0.471	0.113	58.7
Brazil, dried, unblanched		1		1.622	0.236	0.251	4
Cashew, dry roasted		0.2	0.07	1.4	1.217	0.356	69.2
Chia seeds, dried(B2: 1 oz)	36	0.869	0.05	5.817			
Flax seed, dried							
Hazelnut, Filbert, dried, unblanched	67	0.5	0.04	1.135	1.148	0.612	71.8
Macadamia nut, dried		0.35	0.04	2.14			
Olives, black, canned	372	0.003	0	0.25		0.011	
Olive oil(B2: 1 Tbsp)			0				
Peanut oil, roasted(B2: 1 Tbsp)		0.253	0	14.27	1.39	0.255	125.7
Peanut, dry roasted			0.04	71			
Pecan, dried	128	0.848	0.04	0.887	1.707	0.188	39.2
Pine nut, dried(B2: 1 oz)	29	1.02	0.05	3.9			
Pistachio, dried	233	0.82	0.06	1.08			58
Psyllium seed, dried	4023						
Pumpkin seed, dried	380	0.21	0.11	1.745			
Sesame seed, whole, dried	9	0.79	0.09	4.515	0.05	0.79	96.7
Sunflower seed, dried	50	2.29	0.09	4.5			
Walnut, English dried	124	0.382	0.04	1.042	0.631	0.558	66
Walnut, Black dried	296	0.217	0.03	0.69			
Watermelon seed, dried	0	0.19		3.55			57.9
Average	**89.5**	**0.5**		**6.7**	**0.8**	**0.3**	**62.1**

Nutrition--Nuts, Seeds & Oils

	3000mg Vitamin C	1mg=1.35IU 600IU Vitamin E	1500 mg Calcium	3mg Copper	18mg Iron	1g Mag.
Alfalfa, sprouted raw	8.2		32	0.157	0.96	27
Alfalfa, dried	147		899		26	230
Almond, dried, unblanched	0.6	32.41	266	0.942	3.66	296
Brazil, dried, unblanched	0.7	10.26	176	1.77	3.4	225
Cashew, dry roasted		0.77	45	2.22	6	260
Chia seeds, dried(B2: 1 oz)			529	1.66	10	
Flax seed, dried						
Hazelnut, Filbert, dried, unblanched	1	32.29	188	1.509	3.27	285
Macadamia nut, dried			70	0.296	2.41	116
Olives, black, canned	1.3		91	0.251	3.3	4
Olive oil(B2: 1 Tbsp)		16.07	0.18	0.226	0.38	0.01
Peanut oil, roasted(B2: 1 Tbsp)		9.37	88	1.63	1.83	185
Peanut, dry roasted					2.57	
Pecan, dried	2	4.19	36	1.182	2.13	128
Pine nut, dried(B2: 1 oz)	2		17	1.02	6.1	234
Pistachio, dried		7.03	135	1.18	6.78	158
Psyllium seed, dried			334		20	51
Pumpkin seed, dried	173		43	1.387	14.97	535
Sesame seed, whole, dried		3.06	975	4.08	14.55	351
Sunflower seed, dried			116	1.752	6.77	354
Walnut, English dried	3.2	3.54	94	1.387	2.44	169
Walnut, Black dried			58	1.02	3.07	202
Watermelon seed, dried			54		7.28	515

	10mg Manganese	600mg Phosphorus	2000mg Potassium	Sodium	50mg Zinc
Alfalfa, sprouted raw	0.188	70	79	6	0.92
Alfalfa, dried	2.53	150	1200	17	0.005
Almond, dried, unblanched	2.273	520	732	11	2.92
Brazil, dried, unblanched	0.774	600	600	2	4359
Cashew, dry roasted		490	565	16	5.6
Chia seeds, dried(B2: 1 oz)		604			5.32
Flax seed, dried					
Hazelnut, Filbert, dried, unblanched	2.016	312	445	3	2.4
Macadamia nut, dried		136	368	5	1.71
Olives, black, canned	0.02	3	9	885	0.22
Olive oil(B2: 1 Tbsp)		1.22		0.04	0.06
Peanut oil, roasted(B2: 1 Tbsp)	2.062	517	682	433	6.63
Peanut, dry roasted					
Pecan, dried	4.506	291	392	1	5.47
Pine nut, dried(B2: 1 oz)		271	613	38	4.26
Pistachio, dried	0.327	503	1093	6	1.34
Psyllium seed, dried	1.6	63	811	54	2.1
Pumpkin seed, dried		1174	807	18	7.46
Sesame seed, whole, dried	2.46	629	468	11	7.75
Sunflower seed, dried	2.02	705	689	3	5.06
Walnut, English dried	2.898	317	502	10	2.73
Walnut, Black dried	4.271	464	524	1	3.42
Watermelon seed, dried		755	648	99	

Nutrition--Vegetables

Nutrients per 100g edible portion

Vegetable	2 Typical Weight(g)	Qty/ 100g	cups or each Volume/ 100g	Calories	g Protein	g Fat	35 g Fiber
Artichoke,Globe	364			50	3.48	0.16	1.25
Artichoke,Jerusalem				76	2	0.01	0.8
Asparagus,cooked				24	2.59	0.31	0.83
Avocado,California	224			177	2.11	17.33	2.11
Avocado,Florida	224			112	1.59	8.87	2.11
Bamboo shoots				27	2.6	0.3	0.7
Bean,green/snap				31	1.82	0.12	1.1
Beet,root				44	1.48	0.14	0.8
Beet greens				19	1.82	0.06	1.3
Broccoli (1 head)	448			28	2.98	0.35	1.11
Brussels sprouts,cooked				39	2.55	0.51	1.37
Burdock root,cooked				88	2.09	0.14	1.83
Cabbage,green (1 head)	1120			24	1.21	0.18	0.8
Cabbage,red, head	896		7/8 cup	27	1.39	0.26	1
Cabbage,savoy, head	672			27	2	0.1	0.8
Carrot 8.5"	107	0.93		43	1.03	0.19	1.04
Cauliflower, head	1232			24	1.99	0.18	0.85
Celeriac	672			39	1.5	0.3	1.3
Celery	896			16	0.75	0.14	0.8
Chinese Cabbage,Bok Choy	896			13	1.5	0.2	0.6
Collards, per stalk	21			31	1.57	0.22	0.57
Corn,cooked			3/4 cup	108	3.32	1.28	0.6
Cucumber	440	0.23		13	0.54	0.13	0.6
Eggplant,cooked				28	0.83	0.23	0.97
Fennel,raw bulb	224			31	1.24	0.2	
Kale,blue				50	3.3	0.7	1.5
Kale,Scotch				42	2.8	0.6	1.23
Kohlrabi				27	1.7	0.1	1
Lettuce,Arugula				25	2.58	0.66	
Lettuce,Belgian Endive				15	1	0.1	
Lettuce,Bibb/Boston				13	1.29	0.22	
Lettuce,curly leaf Endive				17	1.25	0.2	0.9
Lettuce,Escarole				20	1.7	0.1	0.9
Lettuce,Loose-leaf				18	1.3	0.3	0.7
Lettuce,Radicchio				23	1.43	0.25	
Lettuce, Romaine				16	1.62	0.2	0.7
Mushrooms,common	23	4.35		25	2.09	0.42	0.75
Mushrooms,Shiitake				296	9.58	0.99	11.5
Mushrooms,Shiitake,cooked				55	1.56	0.22	1.966
Mustard greens				26	2.7	0.2	1.1
Okra,cooked				32	1.87	0.17	0.9
Onion	176	0.57		38	1.16	0.16	0.59
Parsnip				75	1.2	0.3	2
Pea				81	5.42	0.4	2.21
Peppers,bell 3"	178	0.56		27	0.95	0.2	0.44
Peppers,hot chili				40	2	0.2	1.8
Potato,baked w/skin				109	2.3	0.1	0.66
Pumpkin				26	1	0.1	1.1
Radish,small red				17	0.6	0.54	0.54
Radish,Daikon				18	0.6	0.1	0.64
Radish,Icicle				14	1.1	0.1	0.7

Nutrition--Vegetables

	Typical Weight(g)	Qty/ 100g	cups/each Vol/100g	Calories	g Protein	g Fat	35 g Fiber
Radish sprouts				41	3.81	2.53	
Salsify,cooked				68	2.73	0.17	1.49
Sea Vegetables,Dulse,dried					13.3		
Sea Veg: Irish Moss (Carrageenan)				49	1.51	0.16	
Se Veg.,Kombu				43	1.68	0.56	1.33
Sea Veg.,Nori				35	5.81	0.28	0.27
Sea Veg,Wakame				45	3.03	0.64	0.54
Spinach				22	2.86	0.35	0.89
Sprouts,alfalfa,raw				29	3.99	0.69	1.64
Sprouts,mung,raw				30	3.04	0.18	0.81
Summer squash,Chayote				24	0.9	0.3	0.7
Summmer squash,crookneck				19	0.94	0.24	0.55
Summer squash,Pattypan				18	1.2	0.2	0.55
Summer squash,Spaghetti,cooked				29	0.66	0.26	1.4
Summer squash,zucchini, 8.5"	304		0.33	14	1.16	0.14	0.45
Winter squash,Acorn,cooked				56	1.12	0.14	1.96
Winter squash,Butternut,cooked				40	0.9	0.09	1.26
Winter squash,Hubbard,cooked				50	2.48	0.62	1.74
Sweet potato, 6.5"	190		0.53	50	1.65	0.3	0.85
Swiss Chard				19	1.8	0.2	0.8
Taro,chips				477	2.04	25.47	1.18
Tomato	230		0.43	21	0.85	0.33	0.65
Tomato,sun-dried,oil-packed				213	5.06	14.08	
Turnip,root				27	0.9	0.1	0.9
Turnip greens,cooked,w/o stem				20	1.14	0.23	0.61
Water chestnut,Chinese,raw				106	1.4	0.1	0.8
Water chestnut,canned w/liquid				50	0.88	0.06	0.58
Watercress				11	2.3	0.1	0.7
Yam,w/o skin				118	1.53	0.17	

Vegetable	10,000IU Vitamin A	50mg B1	50mg B2	100mg B3 Niacin	100mg Pant.Acid	50mg B6	800mcg Folic Acid
Artichoke,Globe	177	0.065	0.066	1	0.342	0.11	51
Artichoke,Jerusalem	20	0.2	0.06	1.3			
Asparagus,cooked	539	0.123	0.126	1.082		0.122	146
Avocado,California	612	0.108	0.122	1.921	0.971	0.28	65.5
Avocado,Florida	612	0.108	0.122	1.921	0.971	0.28	53.3
Bamboo shoots	20	0.15	0.07	0.6			
Bean,green/snap	668	0.084	0.105	0.752	0.094	0.074	36.5
Beet,root	20	0.05	0.02	0.4	0.15	0.046	92.6
Beet greens	6100	0.1	0.22	0.4	0.25	0.106	
Broccoli (1 head)	3000	0.065	0.119	0.638	0.535	0.159	71
Brussels sprouts,cooked	719	0.107	0.08	0.607	0.252	0.178	60
Burdock root,cooked	0	0.039	0.058	0.32			
Cabbage,green (1 head)	126	0.05	0.03	0.3	0.14	0.095	56.7
Cabbage,red, head	40	0.05	0.03	0.3	0.324	0.21	20.7
Cabbage,savoy, head	1000	0.07	0.03	0.3		0.19	
Carrot 8.5"	29129	0.097	0.059	0.928	0.197	0.147	14
Cauliflower, head	16	0.076	0.057	0.633	0.141	0.231	66.1
Celeriac	0	0.05	0.06	0.7		0.165	

Nutrition--Vegetables

	10,000IU Vitamin A	50mg B1	50mg B2	100mg B3 Niacin	100mg Pant.Acid	50mg B6	800mcg Folate
Celery	134	0.046	0.045	0.323	0.186	0.087	28
Chinese Cabbage,Bok Choy	3000	0.04	0.07	0.5			
Collards, per stalk	3330	0.029	0.064	0.374	0.064	0.067	12
Corn,cooked	217	0.215	0.072	1.614	0.878	0.06	46.4
Cucumber	45	0.03	0.02	0.3	0.25	0.052	13.9
Eggplant,cooked	64	0.076	0.02	0.6	0.075	0.086	14.4
Fennel,raw bulb		0.01	0.032	0.64	0.232	0.047	27
Kale,blue	8900	0.11	0.13	1	0.091	0.271	29.3
Kale,Scotch	3100	0.07	0.06	1.3	0.076	0.227	
Kohlrabi	36	0.05	0.02	0.4	0.165	0.15	
Lettuce,Arugula	2373	0.044	0.086	0.305	0.437	0.073	97
Lettuce,Belgian Endive	0	0.07	0.14	0.5		0.045	
Lettuce,Bibb/Boston	970	0.06	0.06	0.3			73.3
Lettuce,curly leaf Endive	2050	0.08	0.075	0.4	0.9	0.02	142
Lettuce,Escarole	3300	0.07	0.14	0.5			
Lettuce,Loose-leaf	1900	0.05	0.08	0.4	0.2	0.055	
Lettuce,Radicchio	27	0.016	0.028	0.255	0.269	0.057	60
Lettuce, Romaine	2600	0.1	0.1	0.5			135.7
Mushrooms,common	0	0.102	0.449	4.116	2.2	0.097	21.1
Mushrooms,Shiitake	0	0.3	1.27	14.1			
Mushrooms,Shiitake,cooked	0	0.037	0.17	1.5			
Mustard greens	5300	0.08	0.11	0.8	0.21		
Okra,cooked	575	0.132	0.055	0.871	0.213	0.187	45.7
Onion	0	0.042	0.02	0.148	0.106	0.116	19
Parsnip	0	0.09	0.05	0.7	0.6	0.09	66.8
Pea	640	0.266	0.132	2.09	0.104	0.169	65
Peppers,bell 3"	238-5700	0.047	0.028	0.7	0.12	0.205	24
Peppers,hot chili	770-10750	0.09	0.09	0.95	0.061	0.278	23.4
Potato,baked w/skin		0.107	0.033	1.645	0.555	0.347	11
Pumpkin	1600	0.05	0.11	0.6			
Radish,small red	8	0.005	0.045	0.3	0.088	0.071	27
Radish,Daikon	0	0.02	0.02	0.2			
Radish,Icicle	0	0.03	0.02	0.3	0.184	0.075	14
Radish sprouts	391	0.102	0.103	2.853	0.733	0.285	94.7
Salsify,cooked	0	0.056	0.173	0.392			
Sea Vegetables,Dulse,dried	8010	0.16	0.11	3.2			
Sea Veg: Irish Moss (Carrageenan)		0.015	0.466	0.593	0.176		
Sea Veg.,Kombu	116	0.05	0.15	0.47			180
Sea Veg.,Nori	5202	0.098	0.446	1.47		0.159	
Sea Veg,Wakame	360	0.06	0.23	1.6			
Spinach	6715	0.078	0.189	0.724	0.065	0.195	194.4
Sprouts,alfalfa,raw	155	0.076	0.126	0.481	0.563	0.034	36
Sprouts,mung,raw	21	0.084	0.124	0.749	0.38	0.088	60.8
Summer squash,Chayote	56	0.03	0.04	0.5	0.483		
Summmer squash,crookneck	338	0.052	0.043	0.454	0.102	0.109	22.9
Summer squash,Pattypan	110	0.07	0.03	0.6	0.102	0.109	30.1
Summer squash,Spaghetti,cooked	110	0.038	0.022	0.81	0.355	0.099	8
Summer squash,zucchini, 8.5"	340	0.07	0.03	0.4	0.083	0.089	22.1
Winter squash,Acorn,cooked	428	0.167	0.013	0.881	0.504	0.194	18.7
Winter squash,Butternut,cooked	7001	0.072	0.017	0.969	0.359	0.124	19.2
Winter squash,Hubbard,cooked	6035	0.074	0.047	0.558	0.447	0.172	16.2
Sweet potato, 6.5"	20063	0.066	0.147	0.674	0.591	0.257	13.8
Swiss Chard	3300	0.04	0.09	0.4	0.172		

Nutrition--Vegetables

	10,000IU Vitamin A	50mg B1	50mg B2	100mg B3 Niacin	100mg Pant.Acid	50mg B6	800mcg Folate
Taro,chips	0	0.053	0.029	0.04			
Tomato	623	0.059	0.048	0.628	0.247	0.08	15
Tomato,sun-dried,oil-packed	1286	0.193	0.383	3.63	0.479	0.319	23
Turnip,root	0	0.04	0.03	0.4	0.2	0.09	14.5
Turnip greens,cooked,w/o stem	5498	0.045	0.072	0.411	0.274	0.18	118.4
Water chestnut,Chinese,raw	0	0.14	0.2	1			
Water chestnut,canned w/liquid	4	0.011	0.024	0.36			
Watercress	4700	0.09	0.12	0.2	0.31	0.129	
Yam,w/o skin	0	0.112	0.032	0.758	0.314	0.293	23

Vit. D: 40 IU=1 mcg
Vit. E: 1mg=1.35IU

Vegetable	300mcg B12	3000mg Vit. C	400IU Vit. D	600IU Vit. E	1500 mg Calcium	3mg Cpr	18mg Iron
Artichoke,Globe		10			45	0.233	1.29
Artichoke,Jerusalem		4			14		3.4
Asparagus,cooked		10.8			20	0.112	0.73
Avocado,California		7.9		1.809	11	0.266	1.18
Avocado,Florida		7.9			11	0.251	0.53
Bamboo shoots		4			13		0.5
Bean,green/snap		16.5		0.027	37	0.069	10.4
Beet,root		11			16	0.083	0.91
Beet greens		30		2.025	119	0.191	3.3
Broccoli (1 head)		93.2		0.621	48	0.045	0.88
Brussels sprouts,cooked		62		1.1475	36	0.083	1.2
Burdock root,cooked					49		0.77
Cabbage,green (1 head)		47.3		2.2545	47	0.023	0.56
Cabbage,red, head		57			51	0.097	0.49
Cabbage,savoy, head		31			35		0.4
Carrot 8.5"		9.3		0.594	27	0.047	0.5
Cauliflower, head		71.5		0.0405	29	0.032	0.58
Celeriac		8			43		0.7
Celery		7		0.486	40	0.034	0.4
Chinese Cabbage,Bok Choy		45			105		0.8
Collards, per stalk		23.3			29	0.039	0.19
Corn,cooked		6.2			2	0.053	0.61
Cucumber		4.7		0.2025	14	0.04	0.28
Eggplant,cooked		1.3			6	0.108	0.35
Fennel,raw bulb		12			49	0.066	
Kale,blue		120			135	0.29	1.7
Kale,Scotch		130			205	0.243	3
Kohlrabi		62			24		0.4
Lettuce,Arugula					160	0.076	
Lettuce,Belgian Endive		10					0.5
Lettuce,Bibb/Boston		8				0.023	0.3
Lettuce,curly leaf Endive		6.5			52	0.099	0.83
Lettuce,Escarole		10			81		1.7
Lettuce,Loose-leaf		18			68		1.4
Lettuce,Radicchio		8			19	0.341	
Lettuce, Romaine		24			36		1.1
Mushrooms,common		3.5		0.108	5	0.492	1.24
Mushrooms,Shiitake		3.5			11		1.72
Mushrooms,Shiitake,cooked		0.3			3		0.44
Mustard greens		70		2.7	103		1.46

Nutrition--Vegetables

	300mcg B12	3000mg Vit. C	400IU Vit. D	600IU Vitamin E	1500 mg Calcium	3mg Cpr	18mg Iron
Okra,cooked		16.3			63	0.086	0.45
Onion		6.4		0.4185	20	0.06	0.22
Parsnip		17		1.35	36	0.12	0.59
Pea		40		0.1755	25	0.176	1.47
Peppers,bell 3"		140		0.918	10	0.08	0.46
Peppers,hot chili		242.5			18	0.174	1.2
Potato,baked w/skin		12.9			10	0.305	1.36
Pumpkin		9		1.35	21		0.8
Radish,small red		22.8			21	0.04	0.29
Radish,Daikon		22			27		0.4
Radish,Icicle		29			27		0.8
Radish sprouts		28.9			51	0.12	0.86
Salsify,cooked		4.6			17		0.55
Sea Vegetables,Dulse,dried		12			632		79.2
Sea Veg: Irish Moss (Carrageenan)					72	0.149	8.9
Se Veg.,Kombu				1.1745	168	0.13	2.85
Sea Veg.,Nori		39			70	0.264	1.8
Sea Veg,Wakame		3			150	0.284	2.18
Spinach		28.1		2.538	99	0.13	2.71
Sprouts,alfalfa,raw		8.2			32		0.96
Sprouts,mung,raw		13.2			13		0.91
Summer squash,Chayote		11			19		0.4
Summmer squash,crookneck		8.4			21	0.102	0.48
Summer squash,Pattypan		18			19	0.102	0.4
Summer squash,Spaghetti,cooked		3.5			21	0.035	0.34
Summer squash,zucchini, 8.5"		9			15	0.057	0.42
Winter squash,Acorn,cooked		10.8			44	0.086	0.93
Winter squash,Butternut,cooked		15.1			41	0.065	0.6
Winter squash,Hubbard,cooked		9.5			17	0.045	0.47
Sweet potato, 6.5"		22.7		6.156	22	0.169	0.59
Swiss Chard		30			51		1.8
Taro,chips					45		1.35
Tomato		19.1		0.459	5	0.074	0.45
Tomato,sun-dried,oil-packed		101.8			47	0.473	
Turnip,root		21			30		0.3
Turnip greens,cooked,w/o stem		27.4			137	0.253	0.8
Water chestnut,Chinese,raw		4			11		0.6
Water chestnut,canned w/liquid		1.3			4		0.87
Watercress		43		1.35	120		0.2
Yam,w/o skin		17.1			17	0.178	0.54

Nutrition--Vegetables

Vegetable	1g Mag.	10mg Mang.	600mg Phosph.	2000mg Potassium	Sodium	50mg Zinc
Artichoke, Globe	60	0.259	86	354	95	0.49
Artichoke, Jerusalem	17	0.06	78			
Asparagus, cooked	10	0.152	54	160	11	0.42
Avocado, California	41	0.244	42	634	12	0.42
Avocado, Florida	34	0.17	39	488	5	0.42
Bamboo shoots	3		59	533	4	
Bean, green/snap	25	0.214	38	209	6	0.24
Beet, root	21	0.352	48	324	72	0.37
Beet greens	72		40	547	201	0.38
Broccoli (1 head)	25	0.229	66	325	27	0.4
Brussels sprouts, cooked	20	0.227	56	317	21	0.33
Burdock root, cooked	39		93	360	4	
Cabbage, green (1 head)	15	0.159	23	246	18	0.18
Cabbage, red, head	15	0.18	42	206	11	0.21
Cabbage, savoy, head	28		42	230	28	
Carrot 8.5"	15	0.142	44	323	35	0.2
Cauliflower, head	14	0.203	46	355	15	0.18
Celeriac	20		115	300	100	
Celery	11	0.102	25	287	87	0.13
Chinese Cabbage, Bok Choy	19		37	252	65	
Collards, per stalk	9	0.276	10	169	20	0.13
Corn, cooked	32	0.194	103	249	17	0.48
Cucumber	11	0.061	17	149	2	0.23
Eggplant, cooked	13	0.136	22	248	4	0.15
Fennel, raw bulb	17	0.191	50	414	52	0.2
Kale, blue	34	0.774	56	447	43	0.44
Kale, Scotch	88	0.648	62	450	70	0.37
Kohlrabi	19		46	350	20	
Lettuce, Arugula	47	0.321	52	369	27	0.47
Lettuce, Belgian Endive	13		21	182	7	
Lettuce, Bibb/Boston		0.133		257	5	0.17
Lettuce, curly leaf Endive	15	0.42	28	314	22	0.79
Lettuce, Escarole			54	294	14	
Lettuce, Loose-leaf	11		25	264	9	
Lettuce, Radicchio	13	0.138	40	302	22	0.62
Lettuce, Romaine	6		45	290	8	
Mushrooms, common	10	0.112	104	370	4	0.73
Mushrooms, Shiitake	132		294	1534	13	
Mushrooms, Shiitake, cooked	14		29	117	4	
Mustard greens	32		43	354	25	
Okra, cooked	57	0.91	56	322	5	0.55
Onion	10	0.137	33	157	3	0.19
Parsnip	29	0.56	71	375	10	0.59
Pea	33	0.41	108	244	5	1.24
Peppers, bell 3"	11	0.116	22	199	2	0.14
Peppers, hot chili	25	0.237	46	340	7	0.3
Potato, baked w/skin	27	0.229	57	418	8	0.32
Pumpkin	12		44	340	1	
Radish, small red	9	0.07	18	232	24	0.3
Radish, Daikon	16		23	227	21	
Radish, Icicle	9		28	280	16	
Radish sprouts	44	0.26	113	86	6	0.56
Salsify, cooked	18		56	283	16	

Nutrition--Vegetables

	1g Mag.	10mg Mang.	600mg Phosph.	2000mg Potassium	Sodium	50mg Zinc
Sea Vegetables,Dulse,dried	593	3.7	386	2270	9917	3.9
Sea Veg: Irish Moss (Carrageenan)		0.37	157	63	67	1.95
Se Veg.,Kombu	121	0.2	42	89	233	1.23
Sea Veg.,Nori	2	0.988	58	356	48	1.05
Sea Veg,Wakame	107	1.4	80	50	872	0.38
Spinach	79	0.897	49	558	79	0.53
Sprouts,alfalfa,raw	27		70	79	6	0.92
Sprouts,mung,raw	21		54	149	6	0.41
Summer squash,Chayote	14		26	150	4	
Summmer squash,crookneck	21	0.157	32	212	2	0.29
Summer squash,Pattypan	23	0.157	36	182	1	0.29
Summer squash,Spaghetti,cooked	11		14	117	18	0.2
Summer squash,zucchini, 8.5"	22	0.127	32	248	3	0.2
Winter squash,Acorn,cooked	43		45	437	4	0.17
Winter squash,Butternut,cooked	29		27	284	4	0.13
Winter squash,Hubbard,cooked	22		23	358	8	0.15
Sweet potato, 6.5"	10	0.355	28	204	13	0.28
Swiss Chard	81		46	379	213	
Taro,chips	84		131	824	369	
Tomato	11	0.105	24	222	9	0.09
Tomato,sun-dried,oil-packed	81	0.466	139	1565	266	0.78
Turnip,root	11		27	191	67	
Turnip greens,cooked,w/o stem	22	0.337	29	203	29	0.14
Water chestnut,Chinese,raw	22		63	584	14	
Water chestnut,canned w/liquid	5		19	118	8	0.38
Watercress	21		60	330	41	
Yam,w/o skin	21		55	816	9	0.24

NOTES

NOTES

NOTES

NOTES

Nutrition--Herbs & Spices

2 Herb/Spice	Std. Wt(g)	Qty/100g	8/16=1/2 cup 12 Tbsp=3/4 c Vol. / 100g	Cal	g Prot	g Fat	35 g g Fiber	10,000IU IU A	50mg mg B1
Agar-agar				306	6.21	0.3	0.7	0	0.01
Allspice,dried,ground			1 1/16 cups	263	6.09	8.69	21.64	540	0.101
Aloe Vera,dried				280	5.7	0.8	17.7	5080	0.08
Angelica(Dong Quai),dried				320	13	1.8	17.2	2010	
Anise,whole herb				337	17.6	15.9	14.6		
Anise,seed			1 cup	7	0.37	0.33	0.31		
Arrowroot,powder				357	0.3	0.1			0.001
bkg pwdr,"Calumet" per Tbsp	14.4	7 Tbsp	7/16 cup	3	0	0			
bkg pwdr+crm of tartar,Tbsp	14.4	7 Tbsp		7	0	0			
baking soda, 1 tsp	14.4	7 Tbsp	7/16 cup	0	0	0	0		
Basil,fresh			2 1/4 cups	27	2.54	0.61			0.026
Borage,raw				21	1.8	0.7	0.92	4200	0.06
Burdock,dried				205	10.6	0.7	7.2	7500	1
Calendula,fresh (marigold)			3 1/8 cups		0.64	33			1
Caper,fresh					19	31			
Caraway,whole seed				333	19.8	14.6	12.65	363	0.383
Cardamom,ground			1 1/16 cups	311	10.8	6.7	11.29		0.198
Carob,flour				180	4.62	0.65	7.19	14	0.053
Cayenne,dried ground				318	12	17.3	24.88	41610	0.328
Celery seed,whole seed				392	18.1	25.3	11.85	52	
Chamomile,German,dried				299	11.5	3.9	7.2	365	0.08
Chickweed,dried				213	21.7	4.8	10.8	7229	0.21
Chicory,raw leaves				23	1.7	0.3	0.8	4000	0.06
Chicory,raw roots				73	1.4	0.2	1.95	6	0.04
Chive,fresh raw			60 12" stems	30	3.27	0.73		4353	0.078
Cinnamon,dried ground				261	3.89	3.18	24.35	260	0.077
Clove,dried ground				323	5.98	20.1	9.62	530	0.115
Red Clover,dried				326	11.5	3.6	9.9	2008	0.42
Cilantro,fresh raw				20	2.36	0.59	0.8	2767	0.074
Coriander,whole seed				298	12.4	17.8	29.12		0.239
cream of tartar,1 tsp				8	0	0			
Cumin,whole seed				375	17.8	22.3	10.5	1270	0.628
Curry powder				325	12.7	13.8	16.32	986	0.253
Dandelion,greens,raw				45	2.7	0.7	1.6	14000	0.19
Dandelion,dried (root)				265	16.5	1.6	8.9	14000	
Dill,leaves,dried				253	20	4.36	11.93		0.418
Dill,seed,whole				305	16	14.5	21.09	53	0.418
Fennel seed,whole				345	15.8	14.9	15.66	135	0.408
Fenugreek,whole seed				323	23	6.41	10.07		0.322
Garlic,raw				149	6.36	0.5	1.5		0.2
Ginger,fresh raw				69	1.74	0.73	1.03		0.023
Ginseng,Asian,dried				274	10.9	1.77	7.2		0.17
Honey,strained				304	0.3	0		0	0
Juniper berry,dried			13/16 cup	341	18.2	5.6	12	2026	0.12
Licorice,dried				268	11	1	8.4		0.21
Maple syrup				262	0	0.2	0		0.006
Maple sugar				354	0.1	0.2	0		0.009
Marjoram,dried				271	12.7	7.04	18.11	8068	0.289
Peppermint,dried				302	24.8	5.4	11.4	39579	1.21
Molasses,regular				266	0	0.1		0	0.041
Molasses,blackstrap(sulph.)				235	0	0		0	0.033
Molasses,sorghum				290	0	0	0.1		0.1
Mustard,whole seed				469	24.9	28.8	6.55		0.543
Nasturtium,fresh leaf				48	1.8	1.2	0.5		0.09
Nasturtium,stalk				350	13.2	8.8	3.6		0.65
Oregano,dried			3 1/8 cups	306	11	0.25	14.96		0.341
Paprika,dried			12.5 Tbsp	289	14.8	13	20.89		0.645
Parsley,dried				276	22.4	4.43	10.32		0.172
Parsley,fresh raw				36	2.97	0.79			0.086

Nutrition--Herbs & Spices

							35 g	10,000IU	50mg
2			8/16=1/2 cup		g	g	g	IU	mg
			12 Tbsp=3/4 c						
Herb/Spice	Std. Wt(g)	Qty/100g	Vol. / 100g	Cal	Prot	Fat	Fiber	A	B1
Pepper,black,whole				255	11	3.26	13.13		0.109
Rose Hips,dried				341	13.3	1.9	30		0.38
Rosemary,dried				331	4.88	15.2	17.65		0.514
Saffron,dried				310	11.4	5.85	3.87		
Sage,dried,ground			3 1/8 cups	315	10.6	12.7	18.05		0.754
Savory,dried,ground				272	6.73	5.91	15.27		0.366
Sorrel,fresh					5.6	1.7			
Spirulina,dried				290	57.5	7.72	3.64		2.38
Stevia,dried				254	11.2	1.9	15.2		
Tamarind,pulp				115	3.1	0.1	5.6		0.16
Tarragon,dried,ground				295	22.8	7.24	7.41		0.251
Thyme,dried,ground			12.5 Tbsp	276	9.1	7.43	18.63		0.513
Turmeric,dried,ground			12.5 Tbsp	354	7.83	9.88	6.71		0.152
Vanilla,cured					2.6	4.7	15.3		
Yellow Dock,dried				284	20.3	4.1	12.2		

Nutrition--Herbs & Spices

Herb/Spice	B2 (50mg) mg	B3 (.1g) mg	B5 (100mg) mg	B6 (50mg) mg	Folate (.8mg) mcg	C (3g) mg	Calc (1.5g) mg	Cpr (3mg) mg	Iron (18mg) mg	Mag (1g) mg	Mang (10mg) mg	Phos (.6g) mg	Potas (2g) mg	Zinc (50mg) mg
Agar-agar	0.222	0.2				0	625		21.4	770	4.30	52	1125	
Allspice,dried,ground	0.063	2.9				39.2	661	0.55	7.06	135	2.94	113	1044	1.01
Aloe Vera,dried		6.4				626	460		4.1	93	0.60	94	85	1.1
Angelica(Dong Quai),dried	0.34	6.8				30.4	282		88	265	2.60	334	1070	
Anise,whole herb							646	0.91	36.96	170	2.30	440	1441	5.3
Anise,seed							14		0.78	4		9	30	0.11
Arrowroot,powder	0	0	0.13	0.005	7	0	40	0.04	0.33	3	0.47	5	11	0.07
bkg pwdr,"Calumet" per Tbsp							241		0	0		83	0	0
bkg pwdr+crm of tartar,Tbsp							0		0	0		0	361	0
baking soda, 1 tsp														
Basil,fresh	0.073	0.9	0.24	0.129	64		154	0.29		81	1.45	69	462	0.85
Borage,raw	0.15	0.9				35	93		3.3	52		53	470	
Burdock,dried	0.34	1.3				8.5	733		147	537	6.00	437	1680	2.2
Calendula,fresh (marigold)						133	3040							
Caper,fresh														
Caraway,whole seed	0.379	3.6					689	0.91	16.23	258	1.30	568	1351	5.5
Cardamom,ground	0.182	1.1					383	0.38	13.97	229	28.00	178	1119	7.47
Carob,flour	0.461	1.9	0.05	0.366	29	0.2	348	0.57	2.94	54	0.51	79	827	0.92
Cayenne,dried ground	0.919	8.7				76.4	148	0.37	7.8	152	2.00	293	2014	2.48
Celery seed,whole seed						17.1	1767	1.37	44.9	440	7.57	547	1400	6.93
Chamomile,German,dried	0.43	15				26.7	672		17	292	5.20	322	1320	
Chickweed,dried	0.13	4.7				6.9	1210		253	529	15.30	448	1840	5.2
Chicory,raw leaves	0.1	0.5				24	100		0.9	30		47	420	
Chicory,raw roots	0.03	0.4				5	41		0.8	22		61	290	
Chive,fresh raw	0.115	0.6	0.32	0.138	105	58.1	92	0.16	1.6	42	0.37	58	296	0.56
Cinnamon,dried ground	0.14	1.3				28.5	1228	0.23	38.07	56	16.67	61	500	1.97
Clove,dried ground	0.267	1.5				80.8	646	0.35	8.68	264	30.03	105	1102	1.09
Red Clover,dried	0.33	13				297	1310		0.035	349	5.90	322	2000	
Cilantro,fresh raw	0.12	0.7				10.5	98		1.95	26		36	542	
Coriander,whole seed	0.29	2.1					709	0.98	16.32	330	1.90	409	1267	4.7
cream of tartar,1 tsp							0.2	0.01	0.11	0	0.01	0	495	0.013
Cumin,whole seed	0.327	4.6				7.71	931	0.87	66.35	366	3.33	499	1788	4.8
Curry powder	0.281	3.5				11.4	478	0.82	29.59	254	4.29	349	1543	4.05
Dandelion,greens,raw	0.26					35	187		3.1	36		66	397	
Dandelion,dried (root)	0.21	3.3					614		96	157		362	1200	
Dill,leaves,dried	0.284	2.8	1.461			37.6	1784	0.49	48.77	451	3.95	543	3308	3.3
Dill,seed,whole	0.284	2.8					1516	0.78	16.32	256	1.83	277	1186	5.2
Fennel seed,whole	0.353	6.1					1196	1.07	18.54	385	6.53	487	1694	3.7
Fenugreek,whole seed	0.366	1.6			57		176	1.11	33.53	191	1.23	296	770	2.5
Garlic,raw	0.11	0.7			3.1	31.2	181		1.7	25		153	401	0.07
Ginger,fresh raw	0.029	0.7	0.20	0.16		5	18		0.5	43		27	415	
Ginseng,Asian,dried	0.18	8					288			48.1	1.90	52.8	243	
Honey,strained	0.038	0.1	0.07	0.024	2	0.5	6	0.04	0.42	2	0.08	4	52	0.22
Juniper berry,dried	0.06	1.2					849		15	93	6.30	90	957	
Licorice,dried	0.16	7				62.6	878		88	965	4.70	79	1140	0.3
Maple syrup	0.01	0	0.04	0.002			67	0.07	1.2	14	3.30	2	204	4.16
Maple sugar	0.013	0	0.05	0.003			90	0.1	1.61	19	4.42	3	274	6.06
Marjoram,dried	0.316	4.1				51.4	1990	1.13	82.71	346	5.43	306	1522	3.6
Peppermint,dried	3.89	11				20.1	1620		60	661	6.10	772	2260	
Molasses,regular	0.002	0.9	0.80	0.67	0		205	0.49	4.72	242	1.53	31	1464	0.29
Molasses,blackstrap(sulph.)	0.052	1.1	0.88	0.7	1		860	2.04	17.5	215	2.61	40	2492	1
Molasses,sorghum	0.155	0.1					150	0.13	3.8	100		56	1000	0.41
Mustard,whole seed	0.381	7.9					521	0.41	9.98	298	1.77	841	682	5.7
Nasturtium,fresh leaf	0.35	1				200	211		1.3			85		
Nasturtium,stalk	2.55	7.5				465	1540		9.5			620		
Oregano,dried		6.2					1576	0.94	44	270	4.67	200	1669	4.43
Paprika,dried	1.743	15				71.1	177	0.61	23.59	185	0.84	345	2344	4.06
Parsley,dried	1.23	7.9		1.002		122	1468	0.64	97.86	249	10.50	351	3805	4.75
Parsley,fresh raw	0.098	1.3	0.4	0.09	152	133	138	0.15	6.2	50	0.16	58	554	1.07

Nutrition--Herbs & Spices

Herb/Spice	50mg mg B2	.1g mg B3	100mg mg Pant.Ac.	50mg mg B6	.8mg mcg Folate	3g mg C	1.5g mg Calc	3mg mg Cpr	18mg mg Iron	1g mg Mag	10mg mg Mang	.6g mg Phos	2g mg Potas	50mg mg Zinc
Pepper,black,whole	0.24	1.1					437	1.13	28.86	194	5.63	173	1259	1.42
Rose Hips,dried	0.72	6.8				740	810			139	4.00	256	827	
Rosemary,dried		1				61.2	1280	0.55	29.25	220	1.87	70	955	3.23
Saffron,dried							111	0.33	11.1		28.41	252	1724	
Sage,dried,ground	0.336	5.7				32.4	1652	0.76	28.12	428	3.13	91	1070	4.7
Savory,dried,ground		4.1					2132	0.85	37.88	377	6.10	140	1051	4.3
Sorrel,fresh						1000	1620			1085		1126	2293	
Spirulina,dried	3.67	13	3.48	0.364		10.1			28.5	195		118	1363	
Stevia,dried						11	544	14.7	3.9	349	14.70	318	1780	
Tamarind,pulp	0.07	0.6				0.7	35		1.3			54	375	
Tarragon,dried,ground	1.339	9					1139	0.68	32.3	347	7.97	313	3020	3.9
Thyme,dried,ground	0.399	4.9					1890	0.86	123.6	220	7.87	201	814	6.18
Turmeric,dried,ground	0.233	5.1				25.9	182	0.6	41.42	193	7.83	268	2525	4.35
Vanilla,cured							1900					70		
Yellow Dock,dried		5.4				405	1000		76	320	14.50	757	1220	

Made in the USA
Columbia, SC
17 February 2023